REFLEXOLOGY

INGE DOUGANS was born in Denmark where she received her reflexology training. In 1983 she started the School of Reflexology and Meridian Therapy and in 1985 she formed the South African Reflexology Society. She gives lectures and workshops on reflexology throughout the UK, Europe and the USA, and runs her own busy practice in South Africa. She is the author of *Reflexology: A Practical Introduction* and *The Complete Illustrated Guide to Reflexology*, also published by Element Books.

New Perspectives

THE SERIES

New Perspectives provide attractive and accessible introductions to a comprehensive range of mind, body and spirit topics. Beautifully designed and illustrated, these practical books are written by experts in each subject.

Titles in the series include:

ALEXANDER TECHNIQUE
by Richard Brennan

MASSAGE
by Stewart Mitchell

AROMATHERAPY
by Christine Wildwood

MEDITATION
by David Fontana

DREAMS
by David Fontana

NLP
by Carol Harris

FENG SHUI
by Man-Ho Kwok with Joanne O'Brien

NUMEROLOGY
by Rodford Barrat

FLOWER REMEDIES
by Christine Wildwood

REFLEXOLOGY
by Inge Dougans

HOMEOPATHY
by Peter Adams

TAROT
by A T Mann

New Perspectives

REFLEXOLOGY

An Introductory Guide to Foot Massage for Total Health

INGE DOUGANS

ELEMENT

Shaftesbury, Dorset • Boston, Massachusetts
Melbourne, Victoria

First published in 1991 as *Health Essentials:*
Reflexology by Element Books Limited

This revised edition first published in Great Britain
in 1999 by Element Books Limited
Shaftesbury, Dorset SP7 8BP

Published in the USA in 1999 by Element Books, Inc.
160 North Washington Street, Boston, MA 02114

Published in Australia in 1999 by
Element Books and distributed by
Penguin Australia Limited
487 Maroondah Highway,
Ringwood, Victoria 3134

Designed for Element Books Limited by
Design Revolution, Queens Park Villa,
30 West Drive, Brighton, East Sussex BN2 2GE

ELEMENT BOOKS LIMITED
Editorial Director: Sarah Sutton
Editorial Manager: Jane Pizzey
Commissioning Editor: Grace Cheetham
Production Director: Roger Lane

DESIGN REVOLUTION
Editorial Director: Ian Whitelaw
Art Director: Lindsey Johns
Editor: Julie Whitaker
Designer: Vanessa Good

Printed and bound in Great Britain by
Bemrose Security Printing, Derby

British Library Cataloguing in Publication
data available

Library of Congress Cataloging in Publication
data available

ISBN 1-86204-665-4

CONTENTS

Acknowledgements

I would like to dedicate this book to all the students of reflexology, past, present and future. Without them, this practice could never have evolved into the respected and effective healing art it is today.

AUTHOR'S SPECIAL NOTE: Throughout this book, the term 'foot massage' is used as a convenient shorthand to describe Reflexology. However, the author would stress that this is a convenience term only and is not a proper technical description of the therapy. Reflexology is not massage as understood in the systematic and scientific manipulation of the soft tissues of the body. Reflexology is the application of specific pressures to reflex points in the hands and feet. Nevertheless we feel massage is a useful shorthand justified in this instance for a general understanding of what is involved.

WHAT IS REFLEXOLOGY?

CHAPTER ONE

Reflexology is a gentle art, a fascinating science and an extremely effective form of therapeutic foot massage. As a therapy, reflexology falls into the realm of 'complementary' medicine. As such, reflexology is considered to be a holistic healing technique that aims to treat the individual as a whole, in order to induce a state of balance and harmony in body, mind and spirit.

Since the time of Hippocrates, health has been defined as a balanced state, and disease an imbalanced state. In our modern society, imbalance is all too often the normal; the demands of the high-speed 20th century techno-generation take their toll on the delicate and intricate human body. The transition from the state of imbalance to a balanced state requires a gentle and harmless healing process – a process seldom found in the chemical drugs and radical surgery sometimes so indiscriminately prescribed by the practitioners of conventional medicine.

ABOVE BY APPLYING PRESSURE TO POINTS ON THE FOOT, WHICH RELATE TO SPECIFIC ORGANS OF THE BODY, WE CAN INFLUENCE OUR GENERAL HEALTH.

The body heals itself – if given the chance. Because this healing power lies within, we should learn to support and nurture it, not suppress it. Reflexology helps us do this by activating the body's natural healing powers and working to re-establish the equilibrium necessary for normal functioning and well-being.

Few people are aware of the fundamental role of feet in health and healing. In fact, few people pay any attention to their feet at all. We wear badly fitting shoes, suffocate our feet in socks and stockings, pound pavements, hike trails and altogether place an inordinate amount of strain on our poor feet.

Although we may be vaguely aware of the important role they play in carrying us through life, few people realize the significant role of our feet in our spiritual and physical well-being. Our feet connect us to the ground and are therefore a connection between our earthly and spiritual life. They ground us both literally and figuratively. They are our base and foundation and our contact with the earth and the energies that flow through it.

ABOVE TO MAINTAIN OPTIMUM HEALTH, WE NEED TO MAKE SURE THAT OUR BODIES ARE KEPT IN BALANCE.

The feet are a perfect microcosm of the body. All the organs, glands and other parts of the body are laid out in the same arrangement on the feet as 'reflections' or 'reflexes' of the body parts. In reflexology, when the reflexes on the feet are stimulated, an involuntary response

is elicited in organs and glands connected by energy pathways to these specific reflexes. These reflexes, when correctly stimulated, can have a profound influence on our state of health.

This microcosmic representation of body parts is also evident in the iris of the eye, in the ear and on the hands. They are, however, easiest to locate on the feet, where they cover a larger area and are more specific.

ABOVE ALL TOO OFTEN WE TREAT OUR FEET BADLY BY SQUEEZING THEM INTO ILL-FITTING FASHIONABLE SHOES.

8

LEFT ACCORDING TO IRIDOLOGISTS, THE IRIS REPRESENTS A MAP OF THE HUMAN BODY.

The feet are also particularly sensitive, due to the abundance of nerve endings present.

Nerves conduct electrical impulses. Imagine these impulses as channels of energy that connect the feet to the rest of the body. When pressure is applied to certain points on the feet, electro-chemical nerve impulses are activated, forming a 'message'. This message passes through 'afferent neurons' (neurons conveying messages to the centre) to a ganglion (a collection of nerve cells and fibres that forms an independent nerve centre outside the spinal cord and the brain). The message then passes from the ganglion via 'efferent neurons' (conveying messages out from the centre to the periphery) to the specific organ, which will then respond. The nerve impulses initiated by pressing reflex areas on the feet might possibly link into the autonomic nervous system, which is primarily concerned with the involuntary action of internal organs, muscles and glands.

9

The goal of reflexology is to trigger the return to homoeostasis – a state of equilibrium or balance. Professional massage on the feet serves to establish which parts of the body are out of balance and therefore not working efficiently. Treatment can then be given to correct these imbalances and thus return the body to good working order. Not only is this form of therapy useful for treating existing ill-health, but it is also effective in maintaining good health and thus preventing illness. Health problems can also be detected early by reflexology and treatment can be given to prevent serious symptoms from developing.

ABOVE A SENSE OF DEEP RELAXATION IS ONE OF THE MAJOR BENEFITS OF REFLEXOLOGY.

One of the most important benefits of reflexology is its ability to induce a state of relaxation. Stress – a major problem of the 20th century – is directly responsible for a multitude of modern diseases and disorders. Stress gradually erodes the body's immune system, and the end result is disease. Reflexology can help reduce the negative effects of stress and helps the body normalize, thereby preventing the development of ill-health.

THE HISTORY OF REFLEXOLOGY

Foot massage has been practised for centuries by many diverse cultures around the world. Exactly where it all began is not clear, but the main school of thought claims that it originated in the East at about the same time as acupuncture. There is little doubt that a strong connection exists between reflexology and acupuncture. Both therapies are considered meridian therapies, which propose that energy lines link the hands and feet to various body parts.

The Chinese were certainly aware of the importance of feet in treating disease. In AD1017, Dr Wang Wei had a human figure cast in bronze on which were marked those points on the body important for acupuncture. When treating the sick, the practitioner positioned the needles in the appropriate areas of the body and then applied deep pressure therapy on the soles of both feet. Concentrated pressure was then applied on the big toe. The feet were used in conjunction with the acupuncture needles to channel extra energy through the body. Dr Wei said that the feet were the most sensitive part of the body and contained great energizing areas.

Apart from the Chinese, other ancient cultures also practised foot massage as a form of therapeutic and preventative medicine. The oldest documentation depicting reflexology treatment was discovered in the tomb of an Egyptian physician, Ankmahor, at Saqqara in Egypt. Dating to around 2500–2330BC, it depicts two men 'working' on the feet of two other men.

Another theory claims that foot reflex therapy was passed down to the Native Americans by the Incas. One Native American tribe – the Cherokee Indians of North Carolina – can attest that they have, for centuries, acknowledged the importance of feet in maintaining physical, mental and spiritual balance. According to Jenny Wallace, a therapist from this clan, 'Working on the feet is a very important healing art and is part of a sacred ceremony. The feet walk upon the earth and through this your spirit is connected to the universe. Our feet are our contact with the earth and the energies that flow through it.'

Modern reflexology developed as a result of the enquiring medical minds in Europe and the US in the late 19th and early 20th centuries. The Germans began to look at physiological reflex action in the late 1890s and early 1900s. They began to examine the treatment of disease by massage and developed techniques that became known as reflex massage.

It is generally believed that Dr Alfons Cornelius was probably the first to apply massage to 'reflex zones'. In 1893, Cornelius suffered an infection. In the course of his convalescence he received a daily massage. The treatment from one masseur, who worked longer on the more painful areas, was particularly effective. Cornelius instructed his masseur to work only on the painful areas. After a few weeks Cornelius' pain had completely disappeared. Intrigued, Cornelius began to use pressure treatment in his own medical practice. He published a manuscript *Druckpunkte* or *Pressure Points* in 1902.

ZONE THERAPY

It is US physician Dr William Fitzgerald (1872–1942) who deserves most credit for establishing the basis of modern reflexology with his 'discovery' of zones and his techniques known as 'zone therapy'. Dr Fitzgerald graduated in medicine from the University of Vermont and spent two and a half years working at the Boston City Hospital. He also practised at hospitals in Vienna and London. While working in Vienna, Fitzgerald probably came into contact with the work of Dr H. Bressler, who was investigating the possibility of treating organs with pressure points.

Dr Fitzgerald noticed that, when treating different patients for the same disorder with a minor operation, some would feel considerable pain while other patients would feel very little. He discovered that those who experienced little pain were able to produce an anaesthetic effect on themselves by applying pressure to areas of their bodies.

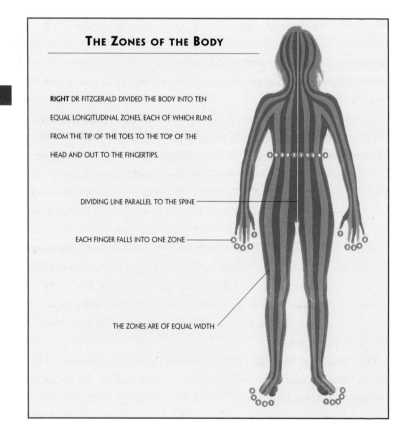

THE ZONES OF THE BODY

RIGHT DR FITZGERALD DIVIDED THE BODY INTO TEN EQUAL LONGITUDINAL ZONES, EACH OF WHICH RUNS FROM THE TIP OF THE TOES TO THE TOP OF THE HEAD AND OUT TO THE FINGERTIPS.

DIVIDING LINE PARALLEL TO THE SPINE

EACH FINGER FALLS INTO ONE ZONE

THE ZONES ARE OF EQUAL WIDTH

Fitzgerald continued his research into this phenomenon while he was working as Head Physician at the Hospital for Diseases of the Ear, Nose and Throat in Hartford, Connecticut. He found that if pressure was applied to the fingers of one of his patients, it would create an anaesthetic effect on the hand, arm and shoulder, right up to the jaw, face, ear and nose. By exerting this pressure on a specific part of the body Dr Fitzgerald learned to predict which other parts of the body would be affected.

ABOVE DR FITZGERALD'S BOOK, *ZONE THERAPY,* REMAINS ONE OF THE CLASSIC WORKS OF REFLEXOLOGY, AND IT IS STILL USED TODAY.

13

Developing this work further, he divided the body into ten equal longitudinal zones running the length of the body, from the top of the head to the tips of the toes. Each finger and toe falls into one zone. These zones are of equal width and extend right through the body from front to back. His theory stated that parts of the body found within a certain zone will be linked to one another by the energy flow within the zone and can therefore affect one another.

In 1917, the combined work of Dr Fitzgerald and his colleague, Dr Bowers, was published in the book *Zone Therapy*. Diagrams of the zones of the feet and the corresponding division of the ten zones of the body appeared in the first edition of this book. The reflex areas, so crucial to modern reflexology, were not singled out for any special attention by Fitzgerald.

The theories of Dr Fitzgerald were not enthusiastically received by the medical profession, but one person believed in his work – Dr Joseph Shelby-Riley. Dr Shelby-Riley, a chiropractor, published several books on the subject, including *Zone Therapy Simplified*

(1919) and *Science and Practice of Chiropractic with Allied Sciences* (1925). It was, however, Dr Shelby-Riley's research assistant, Eunice Ingham, who was destined to make the greatest contribution to modern reflexology.

Eunice Ingham (1879-1974) should probably be referred to as the 'Mother of Modern Reflexology'. It was as a result of her untiring research and dedication that reflexology finally came into its own. She separated the work on the reflexes of the feet from zone therapy in general. Ingham charted a 'map' of the feet that showed the relation between the zones on the feet and their effect on the rest of the body. So successful were her findings, and so effective her treatments, that her reputation soon spread. For over 30 years Eunice Ingham travelled in the US teaching her method through books, charts and seminars to thousands of people both in and out of the medical profession. Her two books *Stories the Feet can Tell* (1938) and *Stories the Feet have Told* (1951) were probably the first books written on the subject.

THE MERIDIANS

Zone therapy is without doubt the basis of modern reflexology and most reflexologists use this as a useful adjunct to reflexology. However, it is my belief that the Chinese meridian system is, in fact, the vital link between the feet and the rest of the body.

According to acupuncture, the body has 12 pairs of meridians. Meridians are pathways through which the energy of the universe circulates throughout the body organs and keeps the universe and the body in harmony. They form the single energy system and maintain the health of the organism. An acupuncturist believes that illness or pain occurs when the pathways become blocked, disrupting the energy flow and breaking the body's harmony. They have developed the use of needles to unblock these pathways. In Shiatsu, the Japanese use direct thumb and finger pressure on the acupuncture points to achieve similar results. In reflexology, finger pressure unblocks the sections of meridians found in the feet.

To date, the majority of reflexologists have believed in the energy lines of the zone system. Although this theory has stood many reflexologists in good stead and contributed greatly to the development of modern reflexology, I personally do not adhere to this theory. I believe that the effects elicited by massaging the feet are caused by stimulation of the six main meridians that run through the feet. Fitzgerald recognized the energy connection between the feet and other body parts, and without his pioneering work, reflexology might not be where it is today. However, as the eastern concept of energy systems was not recognized in the West at the time of his research, the connection with the meridians was not understood. I am convinced that the energy channels linking the feet to the other body parts are the meridians described by the Chinese in acupuncture, and not the zones described by Dr Fitzgerald. This book, therefore, differs from previous reflexology books, because we now move away from the theory of zone therapy and into the realm of meridian therapy.

ABOVE THE CHINESE BELIEVE THAT ENERGY RUNS THROUGH THE BODY VIA PATHWAYS, OR MERIDIANS. THESE PATHWAYS SOMETIMES BECOME BLOCKED LEADING TO AN IMBALANCE IN THE BODY.

WHAT CAN REFLEXOLOGY DO FOR YOU?

CHAPTER TWO

Reflexology is a holistic therapy, and, as such, it aims to treat the body as a whole. It will attempt to get to the root cause of disease and treat this – not just the symptom. In orthodox medicine, the tendency is to hand over responsibility to the doctor and expect him to cure all ills. In holistic therapies, however, much emphasis is placed on personal responsibility. Disease is a direct result of your own thoughts and actions. In order to change this, you have to take a long hard look at yourself – something many people find difficult.

Becoming well requires great effort. We must be prepared to substitute good habits for bad, and become aware of the overwhelming effects that attitude, lifestyle and diet have on health.

It is also important to be willing to 'let go' of disease. A reflexology practitioner will be

ABOVE HOLISTIC THERAPIES, INCLUDING REFLEXOLOGY, WORK ON THE MIND, BODY AND SPIRIT OF AN INDIVIDUAL AND TREAT THE PERSON AS A WHOLE.

kind, compassionate, caring and dedicated to the client's welfare, but no practitioner can decide for the client that he/she is going to get well. That, the client has to do for himself. A genuine desire for health and willingness to let go of disease is of vital importance to any healing process.

Reflexology is not a magic panacea or any kind of instant short-cut. The role of reflexology is to facilitate healing. The reflexologist cannot cure – only the body cures. What reflexology does is work with the subtle energy flows that revitalizes the body so that its own natural healing capacity can get to work. The specific techniques for applying pressure to the feet create channels for healing energy to circulate to all parts of the body.

The human body is a magnificent machine. Thousands of parts work together to keep the body functioning at optimum levels. Unfortunately, the negative effects of attitudes, lifestyle and diet throw the body out of sync, causing malfunctions in various parts. If one part ceases to function efficiently, the whole suffers. Then the minor aches, pains and general fatigue that are often forerunners of more serious complaints begin to manifest.

THE BENEFITS OF REFLEXOLOGY

People of any race, age, colour or creed, men, women, teenagers, children, babies and the elderly – all can enjoy the positive benefits that reflexology has to offer. As reflexology can do no harm, the only restrictions are those determined by the clients'

ABOVE REFLEXOLOGY IS AN EXTREMELY RELAXING TREATMENT, WITH THE POWER TO BENEFIT INDIVIDUALS OF ANY AGE.

pain threshold and their reactions to massage. Elderly people with no specific complaint will benefit from a couple of courses of treatment a year to keep the bodily functions toned and for a sense of well-being. Results are also good with children and babies as they are more relaxed and supple and because their bodies are highly receptive to therapeutic stimuli.

By far the most important benefit of reflexology is its ability to induce deep relaxation. When in a relaxed state, the body has the opportunity to heal itself and function more efficiently. Reflexology can also improve circulation. This in turn cleanses the body of toxins and impurities. Improved nerve supply, revitalized energy and overall body balancing are further positive effects.

REFLEXOLOGY AND STRESS

Stress is difficult to avoid. It is an integral part of 20th-century life – traffic, television, noise, job pressure, family problems, financial problems and global problems such as wars, famines, disease, environmental imbalances, pollution – the list is endless. Today, everyone – young children, women, men and the elderly – are all subject to varying degrees of stress.

Not all stress is negative – it can be immensely stimulating. An athlete or performer subjects him or herself to the stress in order to achieve and experience life's ultimate sensations. The human body is equipped to cope with this kind of short-term stress. However, long-term, constant exposure to stress is devastating. Persistent stress erodes the body's immune system gradually, disrupting the body's delicate chemical and electrical balance. The end result is mental and physical disease.

ABOVE EXERCISE IS A STIMULATING
FORM OF STRESS AND ONE THAT OUR
BODIES ARE DESIGNED TO DEAL WITH.

The stress reaction is a primitive response to a threatening or dangerous situation. It is commonly referred to as the 'fight-or-flight' syndrome. When confronted with a situation we perceive as threatening, the sympathetic nervous system activates involuntary responses designed to activate all the major systems of the body. When the body prepares for 'fight-or-flight', it does so with short-term goals in mind. Fuel is released in the form of glucose or stored blood sugar. More blood is sent to the muscles. Air passages relax and a sense of stimulation is produced. The adrenal glands release adrenaline and noradrenaline into the bloodstream. These two hormones mimic the actions of nervous stimulation in a number of organs in the body. The heart rate increases, blood vessels dilate in some areas and constrict in others, the rate of respiration increases and most digestive activities slow down or stop altogether. These bodily changes prepare us for a short burst of heightened activity.

In modern society many factors can trigger this 'fight-or-flight' response. However, most of these situations cannot be handled with a short burst of activity, and so the body's response is repressed. Stress situations are often continuous, and so the stress responses are on semi-permanent red alert – a situation that cannot be maintained for too long without the body suffering from extreme exhaustion.

Long-term adrenal stimulation, with no discharge of energy, will deplete essential minerals and vitamins from the system, for example Vitamins B and C, which are vital to the functioning of the immune system. This depletion will result in lowered resistance and increased susceptibility to diseases directly related to a lowered immune system, such as ME and AIDS. Long-term adrenal build-up can also affect blood pressure and cause a build-up of fatty substances on blood vessel walls, as well as damage the functioning of the digestive system.

Stress affects different people in different ways and to varying degrees. One person may exhibit cardiovascular problems, another gastrointestinal upset, anorexia, palpitations, sweating or head -aches. Stress can also be linked to infectious diseases. When the

'Fight' Response

THE PITUITARY GLAND RELEASES HORMONES, WHICH STIMULATE THE ADRENAL GLANDS

THE HYPOTHALMUS TRIGGERS THE PITUITARY GLAND WHEN IT RECOGNIZES DANGER

THE ADRENAL GLANDS RELEASE ADRENALIN AND NORADRENALIN INTO THE BLOODSTREAM

RIGHT THE BODY'S NERVOUS SYSTEM RESPONDS TO A 'FIGHT' SITUATION BY RELEASING A NUMBER OF HORMONES.

'FLIGHT' RESPONSE

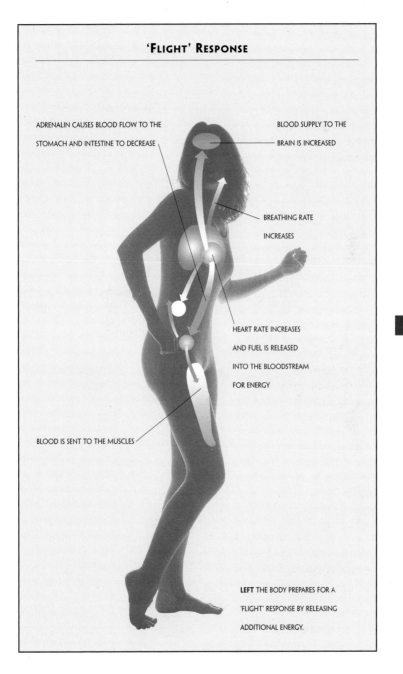

ADRENALIN CAUSES BLOOD FLOW TO THE

STOMACH AND INTESTINE TO DECREASE

BLOOD SUPPLY TO THE

BRAIN IS INCREASED

BREATHING RATE

INCREASES

HEART RATE INCREASES

AND FUEL IS RELEASED

INTO THE BLOODSTREAM

FOR ENERGY

BLOOD IS SENT TO THE MUSCLES

LEFT THE BODY PREPARES FOR A

'FLIGHT' RESPONSE BY RELEASING

ADDITIONAL ENERGY.

body is busy with the effects of residual stress, it cannot organize an effective defence against invading organisms.

Reflexology is a powerful antidote to stress. It helps alleviate the effects of stress by inducing deep relaxation, and thereby allowing the nervous system to function normally and free the body to seek its own homoeostasis.

REFLEXOLOGY AND CIRCULATION

One of Eunice Ingham's favourite sayings was 'Circulation is life, stagnation is death.' Every practitioner acknowledges the importance of good circulation. Blood carries oxygen and nutrients to the cells and removes waste products and toxins from the cells. During this process blood vessels contract and relax. Stress and tension tighten up the cardiovascular system and restrict blood flow. Circulation becomes sluggish, causing high or low blood pressure.

ABOVE REFLEXOLOGY TREATMENT WILL RELAX THE BODY AND REDUCE OUR SUSCEPTIBILITY TO STRESS-RELATED DISEASES.

22

High blood pressure can cause numerous problems – for example arteriosclerosis or hardening of the arteries. Fatty tissues may build-up on the artery walls and blood flow can become restricted. The heart, brain and kidneys may also be affected.

Reduced blood flow to the organs inhibits the oxygen supply and nutrients to the cells. Without oxygen, cells die. Without the proper nutrients, cells fail to function efficiently. The glands and organs begin to malfunction and lose their balancing qualities; this could cause them to overreact or underreact.

By reducing stress and tension in the body, reflexology treatment allows the cardiovascular vessels to conduct the flow of blood naturally and easily.

REFLEXOLOGY AND NERVE FUNCTION

The organs and glands contribute to the overall well-being of the body – each making contributions to maintaining an efficient, fully operated mechanism. But all receive their instructions from the most intricate of all networks, the nerves. These cord-like structures, comprised of a collection of nerve fibres, convey impulses between a part of the central nervous system and other regions of the body. Problems can often be caused by tension putting pressure on a vital nerve plexus or even a single nerve structure supplying a vital organ. As tension is eased, pressure on the nerves and vessels is relaxed, thus improving the flow of blood and its supply of oxygen and nutrients to all parts of the body.

Every part of the body is operated by messages carried back and forth along neural pathways. Stimulation of sensory nerve endings sends information to the spinal cord and brain. The brain and spinal cord send instructions to the organs and muscles. The neural pathways are both living tissue and electrical channels and can be impinged upon or polluted by many factors. When neural pathways are impaired, nerve function is impeded – messages are delivered slowly and unreliably, or not at all, and body processes operate at less than optimum levels. Reflexology, by stimulating the thousands of nerve endings in the feet, encourages the opening and clearing of neural pathways.

23

THE BALANCING EFFECTS OF REFLEXOLOGY

The body is a dynamic energy field; energy circulates throughout the body. For optimum functioning, energy must flow unimpeded and the yin and yang energy

RIGHT FOR A PERSON TO EXHIBIT TRUE HEALTH AND VITALITY, ENERGY MUST BE ALLOWED TO FLOW FREELY THROUGH THE BODY.

currents must complement each other. Reflexology opens up these energy pathways, energizing the physical, emotional and mental aspects of the body. When the body is 'out of balance', it is not functioning efficiently. We are all easily thrown off balance by stress, attitudes, lifestyle and diet. Reflexology helps return the body to a dynamic state of balance.

REFLEXOLOGISTS DON'T....

Reflexologists do not practise medicine. Reflexologists never diagnose a disease, treat for a specific condition, prescribe or adjust medication. They do not treat specific diseases.

However, reflexologists help eliminate problems caused by specific diseases by bringing the body back into a state of balance. Tender reflexes indicate which parts of the body are congested. This 'diagnosis' only relates to parts of the body that are considered 'out of balance' and not specific, named disorders.

THE REFLEXOLOGY TREATMENT

A reflexology treatment should always be a pleasant experience. A client may be tense and apprehensive on the first visit, but any good practitioner will always make an effort to relax the client and give full, undivided attention. The practitioner will ask for a thorough medical history, as all problems, not only those specifically causing trouble at the time, are relevant in building up a complete health picture of the client.

Many people are ashamed of their feet. However, when visiting a reflexologist, any embarrassment regarding the state of your feet should be forgotten. To a reflexologist, your feet represent your body and they tell a thousand stories about the state of your body. Every nick and crevice holds a key to the nature of the problem.

Comfort is the first prerequisite in the treatment, so correct positioning is important. The client will be seated comfortably, preferably on a soft treatment couch. The head and upper part of the body should be upright – the head and neck well supported – so that the client and reflexologist have eye contact. The lower legs will be well supported with the feet in a comfortable position. Shoes and tights must be removed and close-fitting garments should be loosened to allow good circulation.

The practitioner will begin by disinfecting the feet and the first physical contact is usually a gentle stroking movement. The practitioner then proceeds with a general examination of the feet.

Temperature, static build-up, muscle and tissue tone and skin condition are all noted as the therapist tries to get as comprehensive a view of the client as possible. Cold, bluish or reddish feet indicate poor circulation. Feet that perspire indicate a glandular imbalance.

25

BELOW A REFLEXOLOGIST WILL CLOSELY EXAMINE THE FEET FOR ANY SIGNS OF IMBALANCE

OR INFECTION BEFORE BEGINNING ANY TREATMENT.

Dry skin may indicate poor circulation. Callouses, corns, bunions and the like, and their possible links, will also be noted. Any infectious areas should be covered with a plaster or cotton wool before they are worked on as the infection could spread to other areas of the foot and also to the practitioner. Varicose veins should not be worked on as this could cause further damage to the veins. Swelling and puffiness, especially around the ankles, can relate to internal problems. Tense feet may indicate tension in the body; limp feet may indicate poor muscle tone.

WHAT DOES THE TREATMENT FEEL LIKE?

In one word – wonderful. Calming, comforting and exhilarating. It is not ticklish, since the massage technique is too firm to tickle. The foot is always well supported, and the pressure firm but not agonizing.

Sensations vary on different parts of the feet, depending on the functioning of the related body parts. Congested areas will be sensitive – the more sensitive the area is, the more congested it is. The sensations range from the feeling of something sharp (like a piece of glass) being pressed into the foot to a dull ache, discomfort, tightness or just firm pressure. Sensitivity varies from person to person. For example, some people may be relatively unhealthy and have insensitive reflexes, while others may be reasonably healthy and have tender reflexes. This also varies from treatment to treatment, depending on factors such as stress, mood and time of day. In many cases, a client may feel little or no tenderness at all during the first treatment. This does not necessarily mean that there are no congested areas. It more often than not indicates an energy blockage in the feet that needs to be freed. The feet usually become more sensitive with further treatments.

As the treatment progresses, tenderness should diminish. The treatment should never be painful or cause the client any discomfort. The practitioner will adjust pressure to suit the client. No matter what the sensations, treatment is always effective and should leave the client feeling light, tingly and thoroughly pampered.

REACTIONS TO REFLEXOLOGY TREATMENT

People differ, and so do their reactions. On the whole, reactions immediately after a reflexology treatment are largely pleasant – calm and relaxed or energized and rejuvenated. Most people find that they sleep very well following a treatment. However, there is some bad with the good. Reflexology activates the body's healing power, so some form of reaction is inevitable as the body rids itself of toxins. This is referred to as a 'healing crisis' and is usually a cleansing process. The severity of reactions depends on the degree of imbalance, but should never be too radical.

Most common reactions are cleansing reactions that manifest in the eliminating systems of the body – the kidneys, bowels, skin and lungs. The following reactions are common:

- *Increased urination as the kidneys are stimulated to produce more urine, which may also be darker and stronger smelling due to the toxic content*

27

- *Flatulence and more frequent bowel movements*
- *Aggravated skin conditions, particularly those complaints that have been suppressed*
- *Increased perspiration and pimples*
- *Improved skin tone and tissue texture that is due to improved circulation*
- *Increased secretions of the mucus membranes in the nose, mouth and bronchi*
- *Disrupted sleep patterns – either deeper or more disturbed sleep*
- *Dizziness or nausea*

LEFT AFTER A REFLEXOLOGY SESSION YOU MAY FIND THAT YOU TEND TO SLEEP MORE DEEPLY THAN BEFORE YOUR TREATMENT.

- *A temporary outbreak of a disease that has been suppressed*
- *Increased vaginal discharge in women*
- *Feverishness*
- *Tiredness*

Whatever the reactions, however, they are a necessary part of the healing process and will pass. It is a good idea to drink a lot of water (preferably boiled) to help flush the toxins out as fast as possible.

LENGTH OF A REFLEXOLOGY TREATMENT

The length of treatment and number of sessions will vary depending on the client and the condition. For example, the patient's constitution, the history and nature of the illness, age, the ability of his or her body to react to the treatments, the patient's lifestyle and his or her attitude to the treatment – these will all have an effect on the treatment.

The first treatment is investigative and usually takes about an hour. Following treatments are normally 30–40 minutes. If the session is too short, insufficient stimulus is provided for the body to mobilize its own healing powers. If it is too long, there is a danger of over-stimulating, which can cause excessive elimination and discomfort.

Sometimes the first treatment will have an effect. Generally, results are apparent after three to four treatments – either complete or considerable improvement. Long term disorders will take more time to correct than those present for a short time. A course of treatments is recommended for all conditions (even if one session appears to have corrected the problem) to balance the body totally and prevent a

ABOVE THE TIME SPENT ON A TREATMENT VARIES WITH EACH PATIENT AND CONDITION TO BE TREATED.

28

recurrence of the disorder. The course should be 8–12 treatments, once or twice a week. For optimum results, two sessions a week are recommended until there is some improvement in the disorder. Thereafter, the frequency can gradually be reduced.

If there is no reaction after several sessions, the body may be unreceptive. This could be due to external factors, such as heavy medication or psychological attitude, which are blocking the therapeutic impulses. However, as long as reactions are positive there is value in continuing the treatment.

In cases of severe illness such as cancer, multiple sclerosis or paralysis, reflexology may not remove the cause of the disease, but it can significantly improve the patient's general health and promote a feeling of well-being.

PREVENTATIVE THERAPY

Health-threatening dangers lurk around every corner of our modern environment – polluted land, air and water, contaminated and irradiated food, a completely contaminated environment. Add to this the stress of our day-to-day lives – bad diet, attitudes and lifestyle – and we have a potentially lethal cocktail designed to attract disease. Most people wait until disease rears its ugly head before they seek help. However, it makes far more sense to listen to the body's warning signals and take action early. Apart from caring for the body by eating more sensibly, exercising and calming the mind and body through relaxation and meditation techniques, occasional visits to a reflexologist can act as extra 'maintenance' and be of enormous benefit to us all.

29

ABOVE A NUTRIENT-POOR DIET WILL HAVE A DETRIMENTAL AFFECT ON OUR HEALTH.

Preventative therapy is useful for people who have completed a course of treatment and want to avoid any problems re-emerging, as well as for those who may not have any acute symptoms but realize the need for preventative action. Regular treatments can assist the body in maintaining a balanced state, and prevent the possibility of any slight imbalances from becoming troublesome. The intervals between treatments will vary from person to person and may involve weeks or months. For best results, treatment should be applied in the correct manner by a trained therapist, but it can also be beneficial for clients to work on certain reflexes themselves between sessions, to act as a boost to the treatment. To quote Avi Grinberg in *Holistic Reflexology*:

> *'The truly successful treatment is not the one that saves the person from a condition that is in its advanced stage, but is one that prevents its development into a serious or chronic condition.'*

ABOVE REGULAR TREATMENT WILL PREVENT MINOR IMBALANCES IN THE BODY FROM DEVELOPING INTO CHRONIC CONDITIONS.

MERIDIANS

CHAPTER THREE

T he concept of energy channels is a central principle of both reflexology and acupuncture. Both therapies are based on the idea that vital energy is channelled along various lines throughout the body. In acupuncture, these lines are known as meridians; in reflexology, zones. Acupuncture and reflexology both believe that disease is caused by blockages in energy lines, and treatment involves clearing away these obstructions by stimulating various points along the lines. In acupuncture, points situated all over the body are stimulated by needles. The practice of reflexology involves massage on reflex areas and sections of meridians that are found only on the feet.

When Dr Fitzgerald developed the zone theory in the early 1900s, the Chinese concept of meridians was completely unknown in the West. Fitzgerald's 'discovery' of the existence of energy lines was undoubtedly a breakthrough and an invaluable contribution to the reemergence of reflexology in the West. However, it is a logical assumption that the energy lines Fitzgerald stumbled upon were, in fact, the meridians understood by the Chinese for thousands of years.

Closer study of the meridians reveals that the six main meridians are found in the feet, specifically the toes. Thus, massaging the feet can, in actual fact, stimulate and clear congestions in the meridians. When congestions are cleared, energy is able to flow freely and the body is able to achieve a state of balance.

32

The six main meridians are those that actually penetrate the major body organs – the liver, spleen/pancreas, stomach, gall bladder, bladder and kidney. The other six meridians – lung, large intestine, pericardium/circulation, Three E/endocrine, small intestine and heart – are situated in the arms and do not actually penetrate specific organs. However, as the meridian cycle is one continuous energy flow, the six meridians that do not penetrate organs are indirectly stimulated when the main meridians are worked on. This is because the organs related to these meridians are found along the six main meridians. For example, the lung meridian runs along the arm down to the thumb, but the lung itself is penetrated by the stomach meridian, and therefore congestions would be indirectly affected by stimulating the stomach meridian.

Meridians have a long and authentic history. The Chinese discovered the meridian system approximately 3,000 years ago. The fact that this system has been used successfully all this time, and is going from strength to strength, particularly in the West, is proof of its efficacy. It is a logical progression to now incorporate meridians into the realm of reflexology treatment in order to advance and enhance this holistic health therapy.

A basic knowledge of meridians can help reflexologists to understand the disease pathway more comprehensively and be of enormous benefit in pinpointing problems. If, for example, pain, irritation or any other condition does not improve satisfactorily through treatment of the reflex area, one should look at the meridian that traverses the part of the body in question, and treat the reflex area of the organ related to that meridian. For example, a client has arthritis in the little finger, tennis elbow, fibrositis in the shoulder muscles, infection in the lymph glands of the throat, trigeminal neuralgia and hearing diseases. One need simply look at the small intestine meridian that starts in the little finger and ends just in front of the ear and passes the locations of all the above disorders. Could this mean that the small intestine disorder could aggravate or even cause these problems? Clinical results of balancing the meridians certainly indicate this.

33

WHAT ARE MERIDIANS?

All life and matter is energy operating at various frequencies. This energy, known as ch'i or life-force, is what keeps us alive. The Chinese believe that ch'i circulates in the body along meridians, similar to the blood, nerve and lymphatic circuits. This vital life-force controls the workings of the main organs and systems of the body. Ch'i must be able to flow freely along the meridians for each organ of the body to maintain a perfect state of health. If the ch'i is balanced, an individual will be healthy in body, mind or spirit. All illness is a result of an imbalance in the energy flow.

Meridians are located throughout the body. They have been described as containing a free-flowing, colourless, non-cellular liquid that may be partly actuated by the heart (*Handbook of Acupressure II*, by Iona Marsaa-Teergurden). Meridians have been measured and mapped by modern technological methods – electronically, thermatically and radioactively. With practice they can be felt. There are specific acupuncture points along the meridians. These points are electromagnetic in character and consist of small oval cells called Bonham Corpuscles, which surround the capillaries in the skin, the blood vessels and the organs throughout the body. There are some 500 points that are most frequently used. These are stimulated in a

THE MERIDIAN CYCLE

Meridians are classified as yin or yang on the basis of the direction in which they flow on the surface of the body. Meridians interconnect deep within the torso and have an internal branch and a surface branch. It is the surface branch section that is worked as it is accessible to touch techniques. Yang energy flows from the sun, and yang meridians run from the fingers to the face, or from the face to the feet. Yin energy from the earth flows from the feet to the torso and from the torso along the inside (yin side) of the arms to the fingertips. Since the meridian flow is actually one long continuous unbroken flow, the energy flows in one definite direction and from one meridian to another in a well-determined order. Because there is no beginning or end to this flow, the order of the meridian is represented as a wheel. As we go round this wheel following the meridian line, the flow follows this order of the body:

• From torso to fingertips – along the inside of the arm = yin
• From fingertips to face – along the outside/back of the arm = yang
• From face to feet – along the outside of the leg = yang
• From feet to torso – along the inside of the leg = yin

LEFT EACH MERIDIAN IS CLASSIFIED AS EITHER YIN OR YANG.

definite sequence depending on the action required. Meridians are named by the live functions with which they seem to associate. In most cases, this name is the same as that of many of our gross organs.

The Chinese maintain that ch'i circulates in the meridians 25 times a day and 25 times a night. In a sense, there is only one single meridian that goes right round the entire body, but many different meridians are described according to their positions and functions. There are 12 main meridians, which are bilateral (paired), resulting in 24 separate pathways. Each meridian is connected and related to a specific organ from which it gets its name. It is also connected to a partner meridian and organ with which it has a specific relationship. The partner meridians each consist of a yin and a yang meridian/organ and come under the dominance of one of the five elements.

The 12 main meridians control the lungs, large intestine, stomach, spleen/pancreas, heart, small intestine, bladder, kidney, pericardium, 'triple warmer', gall bladder and liver. Within our bodies, the yang organs are those that are hollow and involved in absorption and discharge such as the stomach and bladder; the yin organs are the dense, blood-filled organs such as the heart, which regulate the body. There is constant interaction between yin and yang forces and, if the yin/yang balance between the organs is interrupted, the flow of ch'i will be affected, resulting in ill health.

THE CHINESE CLOCK/ MIDDAY-MIDNIGHT LAW

The Chinese recognized a 24 hour movement of energy referred to as the Chinese Clock. This 'clock' is a 24 hour cycle that divides the day and night into two-hour periods. Each one of these is associated with a surge of energy in one of the organs and its meridian. For example, between the hours of 3 and 5am, the lungs receive their daily booster. (The cycle begins with the lungs and for this reason it is said that these are the hours when it is most suitable to be born.)

CHINESE CLOCK

Organs are stimulated when their energy is 'full', over a specific two-hour period, and sedated in the opposite period of day or night.

3AM–3PM

3am–5am
Lung stimulation
Bladder sedation

9am –11am
Spleen stimulation
Triple burner sedation

5am–7am
Large intestine stimulation
Kidney sedation

11am–1pm
Heart stimulation
Gall bladder sedation

7am–9am
Stomach stimulation
Circulation sedation

1pm–3pm
Small intestine stimulation
Liver sedation

3PM–3AM

3pm–5pm
Bladder stimulation
Lung sedation

9pm–11pm
Triple burner stimulation
Spleen sedation

5pm–7pm
Kidney stimulation
Large intestine sedation

11pm–1am
Gall bladder stimulation
Heart sedation

7pm–9pm
Circulation stimulation
Stomach sedation

1am –3am
Liver stimulation
Small intestine sedation

THE FIVE ELEMENTS

WATER

EARTH

WOOD

FIRE

METAL

The Chinese believe that the best time for stimulating a particular organ is at the two-hour period when its energy is 'full'. Alternatively, it should be sedated at the opposite period of the day or night. For example the lungs should be stimulated between 3 and 5am and sedated between 3 and 5pm. The organ maximum energy periods are included in the detailed section on meridians.

THE FIVE ELEMENTS

Meridian therapy and acupuncture can be more clearly understood in the light of the Chinese belief that five elements – fire, earth, metal, water and wood – comprise the world, and that everything on earth essentially falls into the category of one or more of these elements.

The five elements are generated and destroyed according to a law of cyclical interaction – fire produces earth, earth produces metal, metal finds water, water produces wood and wood becomes fire. By substituting for each element a corresponding yin organ, we see that the heart (fire) aids or reinforces the action of the spleen/pancreas (earth); the spleen/pancreas the lungs (metal); the lungs the kidneys (water); the kidneys the liver (wood) and the liver the heart.

Conversely, just as fire melts metal, metal cuts down wood, wood covers earth, earth absorbs water and water puts out fire, so the diseased or malfunctioning heart adversely affects the action of the lungs, the lungs affect the liver, the liver affects the spleen/pancreas, and the spleen/pancreas affects the kidneys and the kidneys affect the heart. So, to the Chinese people, the nourishing and inhibiting cycle relates not only to the construction and working of the universe, but also to the human body.

YIN/YANG AND THE ELEMENTS

Each of the five elements is assigned at least one yin and one yang organ. Yin and yang are identified with the five elements in the following manner:

Fire:	yin – heart, pericardium (circulation); yang – small intestine, triple warmer
Earth:	yin – spleen/pancreas; yang – stomach
Metal:	yin – lungs; yang – large intestine
Water:	yin – kidneys; yang – bladder
Wood:	yin – liver; yang – gall bladder

From another aspect, the mind fuels the body with negative or positive thoughts. Negative thoughts breed destructive elements. Destructive elements create tension and constrictions of circulation. Disease manifests in tense, sluggish areas of the body. The organs become diseased and fail to function. Our thinking becomes even more disturbed and negative. Pain permeates most of our days, which causes us to become more and more dissociated from nature. Our vital energy becomes weaker and weaker until eventually we die and return to the earth.

SYMPTOMS AND SIGNS TO NOTE ALONG MERIDIANS

Before we look into the meridians and their symptoms, we will take a brief look at the disorders and congestions that can occur along the meridians and indicate where problems may lie. These complaints may take the form of skin disorders, warts, birthmarks, lumps, nail problems and so on.

If a person has skin problems, it may be obvious that the lung and large intestine are the root cause, but note must be taken of exactly where the problem reveals itself on the body, for example, down the legs or on the back. Often these will occur parallel to each other. For example, someone with psoriasis may have it on the outer side of the leg (gall bladder meridian) and down the back (bladder meridian).

Look at the nails for any disorders such as white spots, ridges, problems with the root of the nails or any other nail defects. Ridges on the nails often indicate high acidity, and if you take note on which meridian it manifests, you will see where the congestion occurs – for example, if it is on the thumb, the acidity is congesting the lung meridian. If there are white spots on the nails, these indicate a deficiency of some kind. As the nail takes approximately three months to grow, divide the nail into segments. The centre, for example, indicates approximately six weeks. One can thereby ascertain the approximate period when the deficiency occurred and relate it to the situation at the time – for example, the person may have been on a sugar binge or through a great deal of stress. Always note these signs, and pinpoint the meridian on which they appear in order to trace the problem organ.

THE MERIDIANS

LUNG MERIDIAN

The lungs and large intestine control elimination; the former carbon dioxide, the latter solid residue. As these meridians are partnered, they can directly affect each other. For example chest problems can be accompanied by constipation and vice versa.

The lungs regulate respiration. They are responsible for taking ch'i from the air and for regulating the states of ch'i in the body. Healthy lungs and regular, even respiration ensure that ch'i enters and leaves the body smoothly. An imbalance causes symptoms such as asthma, coughs and various forms of chest congestion. Respiratory functions affect all the rhythms of the body, including the blood flow.

The lungs are called the 'tender' organ because they are the most easily influenced by environmental factors and are involved with regulating sweat secretion, which increases resistance to external environmental influences.

SHOULDER PAIN

STIFF FOREARM

SKIN PROBLEMS

WRIST DISORDERS

NAIL DISORDERS

RIGHT THE LUNG MERIDIAN RUNS FROM THE CLAVICLE DOWN TO THE BACK OF THE THUMB.

LARGE INTESTINE MERIDIAN

The large intestine forms the lower part of the digestive tract and is in charge of transporting, transforming and eliminating waste matter. If these wastes are not eliminated regularly, they can have a toxic effect on the entire system. 'Mental constipation – toxic thoughts and feelings – are often associated with this meridian, in addition to physical constipation or diarrhoea,' to quote from Iona Marsaa-Teegurden's *Acupressure Handbook*.

The *Nei Ching* refers to the large intestine as the generator of evolution and change – and as being integral to the well-being of the whole body. The important function of eliminating waste material is vital to the maintenance of health. If waste is not effectively excreted, the rest of the system has to cope with an additional load of toxic waste and this will cause disharmony throughout the body. An imbalance in the large intestine can result in abdominal pain, diarrhoea, constipation, bloating, swelling, acne and boils, headaches and stuffy nose.

BLEEDING NOSE

COLD SORES

SHOULDER COMPLAINTS

SKIN PROBLEMS

TENNIS ELBOW

ARTHRITIS IN THE INDEX FINGERS, ECZEMA, NAIL PROBLEMS

RIGHT THE LARGE INTESTINE MERIDIAN STARTS AT THE TIP OF THE INDEX FINGER, GOES OVER THE BACK OF THE SHOULDER AND FINISHES ON THE FACE ON EITHER SIDE OF THE NOSE.

STOMACH MERIDIAN

LUNG PROBLEMS

BREAST PROBLEMS

DIAPHRAGM DISORDERS

KIDNEY/ADRENAL
DISORDERS, ALLERGIES

DIGESTIVE PROBLEMS

APPENDIX AND
REPRODUCTIVE
PROBLEMS

THIGH PAIN

VARICOSE VEINS

FOOT PROBLEMS

The functions and activities of
the stomach and spleen are
closely related. The stomach
controls digestion – it receives
nourishment, integrates it and
passes on the 'pure' food
energy to be distributed by
the spleen. The spleen
then transforms it into
the raw material for ch'i
and blood. If the stomach
does not hold and digest food,
the spleen cannot transform it
and transport its essence. They
are interdependent meridians.

According to Chinese
philosophy, the stomach
is related to appetite, digestion and the
transport of food and liquid, but the ruler of food transport and
energy consumption is the stomach's partner – the spleen/pancreas.

BLEMISHES

EYE WEAKNESS

SINUS PAIN

ACNE, BIRTHMARKS

TONSILITIS,
SORE THROAT,
LARYNGITIS, THYROID
PROBLEMS

LEFT AND ABOVE THE
STOMACH MERIDIAN STARTS
UNDERNEATH THE EYE,
GOES UP TO THE TEMPLE
AND THEN RUNS DOWN
THE BODY TO END AT THE
TOP OF THE SECOND TOE.

The two meridians of the earth element work together more closely than any of the others to stabilize the individual. The earth element represents harmony, and if there is no harmony in the stomach, pancreas and spleen, this will affect all the other organs.

The stomach is referred to by the Chinese as the 'sea of food and fluid' as it governs digestion and is responsible for 'receiving' and 'ripening' ingested food and fluids. Without the nourishing activities of the stomach, the other organs in the body could not function. According to Oriental therapists, the stomach is central, physically and functionally, and therefore any problem in the stomach is quickly reflected in the other organs.

If this organ is out of balance, whatever is taken in, be it physical or psychic food, cannot be utilized correctly. Energy depletion – lethargy, weakness and debilitation – are symptoms warning us that the function of this organ is impaired.

SPLEEN/PANCREAS MERIDIAN

A traditional saying that combines the meaning of several references in the *Nei Ching* states that 'the spleen rules transformation and transportation'. It is the crucial link in the process by which food is transformed into ch'i and blood. If this process of food transformation is not activated, nourishment and ch'i are not available for the muscles so they become weak and the lips and mouth become pale and dry. The spleen is traditionally referred to as the 'foundation of postnatal existence'. If the spleen is imbalanced, the whole body or some part of it may develop deficient ch'i or deficient blood.

Physiologically, the pancreas has considerable control over the body's nourishment, since its secretions help digest all the main kinds of food – proteins, fats and starch.

According to the Chinese, 'The spleen governs the blood.' It helps create blood and keeps it flowing in its proper paths. It, therefore, also influences menstruation. The spleen destroys spent red blood cells and forms antibodies that neutralize poisonous bacteria, thus influencing immunity to infection. Another important function of this meridian has to do with the transformation of liquids; the classics say that oedema (swelling from retention of excess fluids) is related to the spleen.

44

BREAST PROBLEMS

UNDERARM COMPLAINTS

ABDOMINAL PAIN

PELVIC COMPLAINTS

MENSTRUAL PROBLEMS

GROIN PAIN, HERNIAS

THIGH PAIN

KNEE PAIN

SHINBONE PROBLEMS

BUNIONS

TOENAIL PROBLEMS

ABOVE THE SPLEEN/PANCREAS MERIDIAN STARTS AT THE TIP OF THE BIG TOE, RUNS UP THE LEG INTO THE PELVIS, THEN UP THE SIDE OF THE ABDOMEN, ENDING AT THE SHOULDER.

PANCREAS REFLEX

SPLEEN REFLEX

HEART MERIDIAN

PAIN IN THE ARMPITS,
SWOLLEN GLANDS

INNER ARM PAIN
AND WEAKNESS,
NUMBNESS,
ANGINA

WEAK WRISTS

STIFFNESS OR
PAIN IN THE
LITTLE FINGER,
NAIL PROBLEMS

The heart and small intestine meridians are coupled. The *Nei Ching* explains their relationship, 'The heart controls the blood and unites with the small intestine. If the heart becomes heated, the heat will converge in the small intestine, producing blood in the urine.'

The classics say, 'The heart rules the blood and blood vessels.' It regulates the blood flow, so when the heart is functioning properly, the blood flows smoothly. If the heart is strong, the body will be healthy and the emotions orderly. If it is weak, all the other meridians will be disturbed.

It is also said that the heart rules the spirit. So, when the heart's blood and ch'i are harmonious, spirit is nourished and the individual responds appropriately to the environment. If this is impaired symptoms such as insomnia, excessive dreaming, forgetfulness, hysteria, irrational behaviour, insanity and delirium may manifest.

ABOVE THE HEART MERIDIAN BEGINS IN THE ARMPIT AND RUNS
DOWN THE ARM TO END AT THE BACK OF THE LITTLE FINGER.

45

SMALL INTESTINE MERIDIAN

ACNE

SHOULDER
COMPLAINTS

TENNIS ELBOW

ARTHRITIS AND
STIFFNESS IN THE
LITTLE FINGER,
NAIL PROBLEMS

The small intestine meridian rules the separation of the 'pure' and the 'impure'. It continues the process of separation and absorption of food begun in the stomach. Because the meridian is in charge of assimilation, this flow has considerable influence over body nourishment and body-mind vitality.

The small intestine influences the functioning of the large intestine both directly and indirectly. In addition to passing solid residue on to the large intestine, the small intestine also controls the proportion of liquid to solid matter in the faeces, reabsorbing some liquids for the body's use and passing some on to be eliminated.

ABOVE AND OPPOSITE THE SMALL INTESTINE MERIDIAN STARTS ON THE TIP OF THE LITTLE FINGER AND RUNS ALONG THE POSTERIOR SIDE OF THE FOREARM. IT THEN RUNS BEHIND THE SHOULDER, ALONG THE SIDE OF THE NECK, TO THE CHEEK AND CORNER OF THE EYE BEFORE ENTERING THE EAR.

EAR PROBLEMS

TRIGEMINAL NEURALGIA

SWOLLEN LYMPH GLANDS

The 'sorting out' process – keeping that which has value and passing on waste to where it can be removed – happens on all levels, both physiological and psychological, for example in sorting out the 'rubbish' from that which is useful in terms of ideas, emotions and thoughts. If this function is not operating efficiently symptoms that express this confusion may arise – for example hearing difficulties, such as the inability to distinguish different sounds. Thus the flow relates not only to assimilation of foodstuffs but also to assimilation of experience, feelings and ideas and to spiritual nourishment.

47

BLADDER MERIDIAN

The partnership of the kidney and bladder meridians is one of the most obvious and means that the bladder meridian has a role in stimulating and regulating the kidneys.

The function of the bladder is to receive and excrete urine produced in the kidneys, and the meridian is therefore in charge of

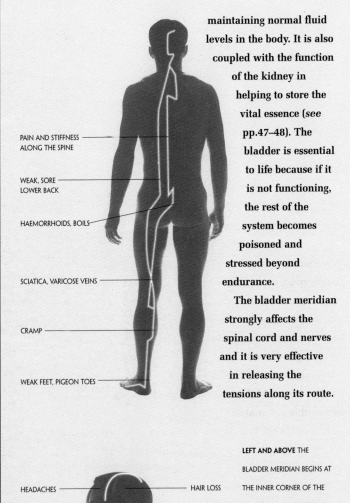

maintaining normal fluid levels in the body. It is also coupled with the function of the kidney in helping to store the vital essence (*see* pp.47–48). The bladder is essential to life because if it is not functioning, the rest of the system becomes poisoned and stressed beyond endurance.

The bladder meridian strongly affects the spinal cord and nerves and it is very effective in releasing the tensions along its route.

PAIN AND STIFFNESS ALONG THE SPINE

WEAK, SORE LOWER BACK

HAEMORRHOIDS, BOILS

SCIATICA, VARICOSE VEINS

CRAMP

WEAK FEET, PIGEON TOES

HEADACHES

HAIR LOSS

NECK TENSION

LEFT AND ABOVE THE BLADDER MERIDIAN BEGINS AT THE INNER CORNER OF THE EYE, RUNS OVER THE CROWN OF THE HEAD, DOWN THE BACK OF THE LEGS AND FINISHES ON THE OUTER EDGE OF THE LITTLE TOE.

KIDNEY MERIDIAN

The *Nei Ching* states, 'When the kidneys are deficient… the spirit becomes easily provoked.'

'The kidneys store the Jing' and rule birth, development and maturation. Jing is the substance – a vital essence – that is the source of life and individual development. It has the potential to differentiate into yin and yang and therefore produces life. The body and all the organs need Jing to thrive, and because the kidneys store Jing, they bestow this potential for life activity. They have, therefore, a special relationship with the other organs because the yin and yang, or life activity, of each organ ultimately depends on the yin and yang of the kidneys.

The kidneys regulate the amount of water in the body. Fluid is essential to life. The flow of the fluid enables waste material to be collected and excreted in the form of urine. Enormous amounts of

LUNG CONGESTION

BREAST LUMPS

SOLAR PLEXUS AND
DIAPHRAGM PROBLEMS

BLADDER WEAKNESS

ECZEMA, SEXUAL
PROBLEMS,
INFERTILITY

THIGH PAIN,
VARICOSE VEINS

49

ABOVE AND OVERLEAF THE KIDNEY MERIDIAN BEGINS ON THE SOLE OF THE FOOT AND RUNS UP THE BACK OF THE LEG, CURVING ROUND TO THE FRONT OF THE LOWER THIGH THEN STRAIGHT UP THE FRONT OF THE BODY TO THE BREASTBONE.

PHLEBITIS ON
INNER CALVES

SHINBONE SORES

SWOLLEN ANKLE

PAINFUL SOLES

blood flow through the kidneys to be purified. If the blood does not flow as it should, symptoms such as high blood pressure or hypertension may result and there may be a build-up of toxic substances that the body would be unable to deal with.

CIRCULATION/PERICARDIUM MERIDIAN

SWOLLEN, PAINFUL
ARMPITS

SKIN PROBLEMS IN
ELBOW CREASE

CARPAL TUNNEL
SYNDROME

HOT PALMS

ECZEMA IN MIDDLE
FINGERS, NAIL PROBLEMS

The pericardium and triple warmer are coupled meridians and both have protective functions. The pericardium protects the heart – the ruler – and the triple warmer protects the other nine meridians. The condition of either affects the other; if the triple warmer is imbalanced, the organs are deprived of proper nourishment and revolt against the heart; if the pericardium is weak, the

LEFT THE CIRCULATION/PERICARDIUM
RUNS FROM THE NIPPLE DOWN THE ARM
TO THE BACK OF THE MIDDLE FINGER.

heart will be attacked and the nourishing activities of the triple warmer will be less effective.

One main function of this meridian is to protect the heart – physically as well as energetically. The pericardium is a fibrous sac enclosing a slippery lubricated membrane that prevents friction as the heart beats. Stresses and shocks first affect the pericardium and do not penetrate the heart unless the pericardium is weakened.

TRIPLE WARMER/ENDOCRINE/THREE E MERIDIAN

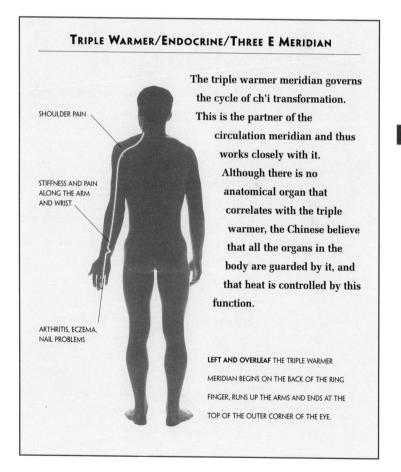

SHOULDER PAIN

STIFFNESS AND PAIN
ALONG THE ARM
AND WRIST

ARTHRITIS, ECZEMA,
NAIL PROBLEMS

The triple warmer meridian governs the cycle of ch'i transformation. This is the partner of the circulation meridian and thus works closely with it. Although there is no anatomical organ that correlates with the triple warmer, the Chinese believe that all the organs in the body are guarded by it, and that heat is controlled by this function.

LEFT AND OVERLEAF THE TRIPLE WARMER MERIDIAN BEGINS ON THE BACK OF THE RING FINGER, RUNS UP THE ARMS AND ENDS AT THE TOP OF THE OUTER CORNER OF THE EYE.

The three 'heaters' or 'warmers' correspond to divisions of the torso; the upper warmer to the thoracic cavity; the middle warmer to the abdominal cavity; the lower warmer to the pelvic cavity. This meridian governs activities involving all the organs.

EYE PAIN

EAR PROBLEMS

It unites the respiratory, digestive and excretory functions into an energetic whole. It may be related to the hypothalamus, the link between the nervous system and endocrine glands. Its functions include:

1   Regulation of the autonomic nervous system and therefore of the heart and abdominal organs, especially in their response to emotion.

2   Control of the pituitary gland (which regulates output of all the endocrine glands).

3   Regulation of body temperature, appetite and thirst.

4   Control of emotions and moods – the urges of pleasure and displeasure that influence social relations.

This meridian, like its partner, has several names, as it is tied to numerous organs. In English it is called the triple warmer, in Chinese *sanjiao,* which means three body cavity, signifying the division of the body into three sections. The burner of the upper section, the breast cavity, is the lungs; the middle burner in the diaphragm section is the spleen/pancreas; and the burners of the lower pelvic section are the kidneys.

GALL BLADDER MERIDIAN

It is essential to note that the Chinese think about the organs as functions operating on all levels of the body-mind ... 'the liver has the functions of a military leader who excels in his strategic planning; the gall bladder occupies the position of an important and upright official who excels through his decisions and judgement' (*Nei Ching*).

According to the Ancient Chinese, the attitudes of all the other organs originate in the energy of the gall bladder. It is different from the other hollow organs in that all the others transport 'impure' or foreign matter – food, liquids and the waste products thereof. Only the gall bladder transports 'pure' liquids exclusively, in that it stores and concentrates bile.

This meridian is one of the most well-travelled meridians, traversing almost the entire body except the arms. It zigzags throughout the head in a pattern that, in times of stress and tension, becomes like a vice and is therefore important in cases of headaches, neck tension and 'uptightness'.

SHOULDER PAIN

ASTHMA

SHINGLES

ARTHRITIS

GROIN PAIN

SKIN PROBLEMS

KNEE COMPLAINTS

CORNS, ATHLETE'S FOOT, HAMMERTOE

LEFT AND OVERLEAF THE GALL BLADDER MERIDIAN STARTS AT THE OUTER CORNER OF THE EYE, RUNS ACROSS THE TEMPLE AND DOWN TO THE SHOULDER. IT THEN RUNS DOWN THE BODY AND LEG TO FINISH ON THE BACK OF THE FOURTH TOE.

MIGRAINES

EYE WEAKNESS

EAR WEAKNESS

NECK TENSION

The *Nei Ching* says that the gall bladder rules decision-making. Thus anger and rash decisions may be due to an excess of gall bladder *ch'i*, while indecision and timidity may be a sign of gall bladder disharmony and weakness.

LIVER MERIDIAN

LIVER PROBLEM

DIGESTIVE PROBLEMS

ECZEMA, FERTILITY AND SEXUAL PROBLEMS

THIGH PAIN, VARICOSE VEINS

KNEE PAIN

SHINBONE, SORES AND PHLEBITIS

PROBLEMS WITH THE BIG TOE

'The liver rules flowing and spreading' according to the Chinese classics. The liver or liver *ch'i* is responsible for the smooth movement of bodily substances and for the regularity of body activities. It moves the *ch'i* and blood in all directions, sending them to every part of the body. The *Nei Ching* metaphorically calls the liver 'the general of an army' because it maintains evenness and harmony of movement throughout the body.

ABOVE THE LIVER MERIDIAN STARTS AT THE BACK OF THE BIG TOE AND RUNS UP THE LEG TO THE GENITAL REGION, FINISHING JUST BELOW THE NIPPLE.

The liver is the primary centre of metabolism. Not only does it secrete bile, synthesize proteins, neutralize toxins and regulate blood sugar levels, it also stores glycogen (starch), changes it back into glucose (sugar) and releases it when needed. Since the brain does not store any glucose, the liver's steady supply is crucial to life, and this is why the Chinese saw the liver as vital to conscious and unconscious thought processes.

The liver meridian helps control the functions of the nervous system and is very important for psychological problems such as depression and anger. Motivation – the will to become 'that self which one truly is'... is associated with balance of this meridian, along with a sense of well-being and a reasonable temperament.

CASE HISTORIES

The reflexologist will require a detailed case history of all symptoms from the client, not only those causing the most severe problems at the time of consultation. These complaints can then be related to the meridians to find out which organs are out of balance. In most countries, reflexologist are not permitted to diagnose any specific condition. Instead of using the symptoms to diagnose a medical condition, a therapist will understand the complaints in accordance with the Chinese philosophy of energy flow blockage.

Study of the path of the 12 meridians shows that the stomach meridian penetrates all the major organs in the body as well as passing through all the reflexes of the major organs in the feet. This is, therefore, the dominant meridian and it is often the root cause of congestions. This will obviously affect the partner meridian, the spleen/pancreas, as well as all the other meridians. This root congestion will manifest as different symptoms in different people, but in 90 per cent of all problems, the stomach and its meridian will be involved.

In the case histories where there are problems with the arms and hands these relate to the lung, large intestine, circulation/ pericardium, triple warmer/endocrine, small intestine and heart meridians. None of these meridians penetrate any of the major organs, but a problem with an organ can cause a blockage in the ch'i energy in the arms and hands resulting in uncomfortable symptoms. It is of vital importance to do a complete reflexology treatment in each case, no matter what the symptoms, rather than to work only on the isolated reflexes that are congested. Weakness may be expressed in congestions of ch'i energy at any point along a meridian, not just in the actual organs. For example, in the case history below relating to the large intestine meridian, the main symptoms were manifest in problems on the arms and face, yet the cause was a large intestine imbalance. The kidney and bladder meridians are partner meridians and the main symptoms that indicate imbalance in these organs are headaches, weak eyes, neck tension and back problems and, to some degree, sciatica and leg problems. Disease in the liver and gall bladder meridians often manifest as migraines, gout, nausea, gall stones, frozen shoulder, hip and leg complaints and sexual problems.

The following case histories have all been effectively treated with the reflexology techniques described in this book in chapter 6. The techniques cleared the congestions in the meridians, allowing the energy to flow freely and the body to reach a state of balance. Each case history has been described so that the reader can relate the most painful symptoms to blockages along specific meridians but, as previously mentioned, one will inevitably find numerous symptoms relating to the stomach, spleen and pancreas and their meridians. Therefore a change to a more healthy diet and lifestyle will always have positive results.

LEFT THE REFLEXOLOGIST WILL BEGIN A SESSION BY TAKING A FULL MEDICAL HISTORY AS WELL AS DETAILS OF ANY CURRENT COMPLAINTS.

CASE HISTORY: LUNG MERIDIAN

FEMALE: Age – 30s

SYMPTOMS: The main reason this client came to me for treatment was severe pain in a 'nerve' in both thumbs.

OTHER SYMPTOMS NOTED: Feels a 'total mess'; allergies; skin problems; rashes on her face and scalp; frequently blocked nose; headaches (forehead and neck); wine makes her nauseous; discontinued contraceptive pills three to four months previously – periods are now regular but heavy and painful; suffers slight constipation.

On studying the case history, I noticed obvious symptoms related to the stomach, spleen/pancreas and their meridians – such as allergies, rashes on her face, heavy and painful periods and slight constipation. But the reason she sought treatment was due to the problem with her thumbs, which indicates a blockage in the ch'i energy of the lung meridian.

57

CASE STUDY: LARGE INTESTINE (COLON) MERIDIAN

FEMALE: Age – 38

SYMPTOMS: As a teenager she had a wart on her right index finger. She suffered from cold sores on the lips and inside the nose four times a year for which treatment was required. Constipation. Nervous stomach that would progress into painful colic if left unattended. Colds invariably developed into chest problems and occasionally pneumonia. As soon as she disrupts her diet she develops fever blisters on her lips and sores in her

nose, and the wart scar becomes sore and itchy. These are all symptoms found along the large intestine meridian and when the sores erupt they are warning signals of overloading this organ.

LEFT STIMULATING THE LARGE INTESTINE.

Again none of the meridians in the arm and face penetrate any major organs. But organs related to the meridians in the arms – in this case the large intestine – are penetrated by the stomach and other meridians and the cause will therefore usually be found in one or more of the major organs and their meridians.

CASE STUDY: STOMACH MERIDIAN

FEMALE: Age – 55

SYMPTOMS: This client came to me with a continuous laryingitis problem that had occurred six times in one year.
OTHER SYMPTOMS NOTED: fatigue; constipation; tension headaches.
PREVIOUS OPERATIONS: Appendectomy; hysterectomy; lumpectomy from breast under nipple.

ABOVE THE STOMACH REFLEX (SHADED AREA) IS FOUND ON THE SOLES OF BOTH FEET

These symptoms all run along the stomach meridian except the tension headaches, which relate to the bladder meridian. The hysterectomy can be seen as caused by a combination of meridians – the stomach and the spleen/pancreas. This is a classic example of a *ch'i* energy imbalance along the stomach meridian. Over the years symptoms have been dealt with by operations and medication. However, the main cause, an imbalance in the acid/alkaline intake in food, had not been considered.

CASE STUDY: SPLEEN/PANCREAS MERIDIAN

FEMALE: Age – late 20s.
SYMPTOMS: Chronic skin problems on the face; system feels 'burny'; constipation; headaches; painful menstruation until she started taking contraceptive pill three months previously.

PREVIOUS OPERATIONS: Bunions removed.

This case showed a combination of problems along the stomach and spleen/pancreas meridians. The bunion problem was an early indication of an imbalance in the pancreas, but, as the cause was not treated, the problems moved on to the stomach, causing skin and digestive problems. The headaches are due to congestions on the bladder meridian.

CASE STUDY: HEART MERIDIAN

FEMALE: Age – 62

SYMPTOMS: Medical diagnosis of a weak heart – has an 'extra tick'; pain in little finger on the left hand; aching muscles on the left side of the body, specifically the left shoulder, which can last up to three to four weeks; middle-ear imbalance. (Refer to illustrations of the heart meridian and its partner the small intestine – pp.44 and 45.)

OTHER SYMPTOMS NOTED: Constipation; nausea that continues at times for up to three weeks; instant migraines after eating cheese or chocolate; high blood pressure; problems with menstrual cycle – still has periods despite her age – and had cramps that stopped when she started taking contraceptive pills.

PREVIOUS OPERATIONS: Appendectomy; bunion removal 20 years before; three cysts removed from the breast.

Although there are numerous problems relating to the heart meridian, I believe the main cause is on the stomach and spleen/pancreas meridians – obvious in the problems with the menstrual cycle, cysts, bunions and appendectomy. The liver and gall bladder are also penetrated by the stomach meridian, which could produce the symptoms of nausea and migraines.

Note also that the kidneys are on the stomach meridian and the heart is on the kidney meridian. To take care of a weak heart, one should not overload the kidneys. This can be prevented by ensuring correct acid/alkaline balance in food intake.

CASE STUDY: SMALL INTESTINE MERIDIAN

FEMALE: Age – early 30s

SYMPTOMS: Severe neck, back and shoulder problems – pinched sensation from shoulder down the arm; at one point she lost all feeling in her arm; weak stomach – often experiences cramps after meals; weakness in throat; tennis elbow; at the age of six she had a hernia in the groin; at the age five years she suffered a severe ear infection that caused balance problems.

ABOVE THE SMALL INTESTINE REFLEX IS FOUND ON THE SOLES OF BOTH FEET.

Problems along the small intestine meridian are obvious in the symptoms on the shoulder, neck/arm, elbow, ears and throat. Again remember that meridians in the arms do not penetrate any major organs and one would have to look for the cause on one of the main meridians and the related organs. The weak stomach and cramps after meals indicate a stomach imbalance. However, the *ch'i* energy congestions are mainly located along the arm, shoulder, neck, ears and throat.

CASE STUDY: BLADDER MERIDIAN

MALE: Age – 50s

SYMPTOMS: Daily migraines that run from the back of the head over the crown; generally feels stressed at work and at home; does not sleep well – the patient has to relieve himself three to four times a night; fatigue.

PREVIOUS OPERATIONS: Appendectomy; tonsillectomy; prostate surgery.

LEFT THE BLADDER MERIDIAN ENDS ON THE OUTER EDGE OF THE LITTLE TOE.

The appendix and tonsils are on the stomach meridian, whereas the prostate is on the spleen/pancreas meridian. Feeling stressed, bad sleep patterns and fatigue are the result of an imbalance on the stomach and spleen/pancreas meridians. The effects – headaches and weak bladder – are found on the bladder meridian.

CASE STUDY: KIDNEY MERIDIAN

MALE: Age – mid 60s
SYMPTOMS: General bad circulation; painful calves; tingling burning sensation on the feet; has to get up every night to urinate.
PREVIOUS OPERATIONS: Three bypass operations; elbow lumpectomy.

61

Reference to the kidney meridian shows that the heart is situated on its pathway. The burning area on the feet was around the kidney reflexes. Furthermore, five plantar warts were situated on the heart reflex of his foot. The lump on the elbow can be traced to the heart meridian. Problems with the calf muscles relate to the partner meridian, the bladder.

CASE STUDY: CIRCULATION/PERICARDIUM MERIDIAN

I have only seen case histories along the pericardium meridian as symptoms within larger case histories. Lesser symptoms such as eczema, psoriasis, pains in the armpits, carpal tunnel syndrome and arthritis in the middle finger have all been periphery problems of imbalances along the stomach, spleen/ pancreas or kidney meridians. Other symptoms that are a result of an imbalance along the pericardium meridian are heart disease, disturbances in heart rhythm, mental disorders such as fear, nervousness and schizophrenia; car sickness and nausea.

CASE STUDY: TRIPLE WARMER/ENDOCRINE/THREE E MERIDIAN

FEMALE: Age – early 30s

SYMPTOMS: Severe eczema on both ring fingers – cannot wear rings; prolapsed uterus – doctor recommended a hysterectomy after a difficult birth.

PREVIOUS OPERATIONS: Tonsillectomy; appendectomy; lumpectomy on breast around nipple area.

All the symptoms and operations are a result of imbalances along the stomach and spleen/pancreas meridians. The effects of the imbalances have manifest as severe eczema on the ring fingers – the endocrine meridian.

CASE STUDY: GALL BLADDER MERIDIAN

FEMALE: Age – 50s

SYMPTOMS: Depression and nervousness; pain in the right knee extending up to the hip joint – mainly affecting her during the night; acidic burning urine; previous kidney problems; headaches on the temple and top of the head; pain around the ears; heavy menstruation although at menopause age; hot flushes; slight constipation.

The client came to me for treatment for depression and nervousness. This can sometimes be seen as an imbalance in the pancreas and is therefore

tied in with the spleen/pancreas and stomach and their meridians. The other symptoms noted – headaches, pain around the ears and pain in the knee relate to the gall bladder meridian. The previous kidney problems, acidic burning urine, heavy menstruation, hot flushes and slight constipation can also be related to the stomach and spleen/pancreas and their meridians.

LEFT THE GALL BLADDER REFLEX (SHADED AREA) IS FOUND ON THE SOLE OF THE FOOT.

MAPPING THE FEET

CHAPTER FOUR

Understanding the structure of the feet in relation to the body is the first and most important step to understanding reflexology. It is, in fact, very simple, as the feet are a perfect microcosm, or mini-map, of the whole body and all the organs and body parts are reflected on the feet in almost the same arrangement as in the body. These reflexes are found on the soles, tops and along the inside and outside of the feet, and their positions follow a logical anatomical pattern similar to that of the body.

MAPPING THE REFLEXES ON THE FEET

The body itself can be considered as divided horizontally into four parts:
- The head and neck area
- The thoracic area from the shoulders to the diaphragm
- The abdominal area from the diaphragm to the pelvic area
- The pelvis

These areas are clearly distinguished on the feet and provide a precise picture of the body as it is reflected on the feet.

1 The head and neck area = the toes
2 The thoracic area = the ball of the foot
3 The abdominal area = the arch
4 The pelvic area = the heel

5 The reproductive area = the ankle

6 The spine = the inner foot

7 The outer body = the outer foot

8 Breast area and special circulation points = the tops of the feet

THE HEAD AND NECK AREA - THE TOES

The toes incorporate reflexes to all parts of the body found above the shoulder girdle. Imagine the two big toes as two halves of your head, with a common neck. Obviously some reflexes in the toes overlap as they do in the body. Each big toe contains reflex points for the pituitary gland, pineal gland, hypothalamus, brain, temples, teeth, the seven cervical (neck) vertebrae, sinuses, mastoid, tonsils, nose, mouth and other face reflexes as well as part of the eustachian tubes.

The other four toes on each foot contain reflex points for the eyes, ears, teeth, sinuses, lachrymal glands (tear ducts), speech centre, upper lymph system, collar bone (shoulder girdle), eustachian tubes, 'chronic' eye and ear problems.

THE HEAD AND THE BRAIN

Reflexes of the head and the brain can be found on the pads of the big toes, from the tip behind the nail down over the metatarsal bone. Reflexes for the sides of the head and brain are on the sides of the big toes. On the top of the toes are the face reflexes including the mouth, nose, teeth and tonsils. The neck reflexes are at the base of the big toe.

THE SINUSES

The sinuses are cavities within the skull bones situated above and to the sides of the nose in the cheekbones behind the eyebrows. They communicate with the nasal cavities through small openings. They act as protection for the eyes and the brain and give resonance to the voice. The reflexes are situated on the tips of all the toes.

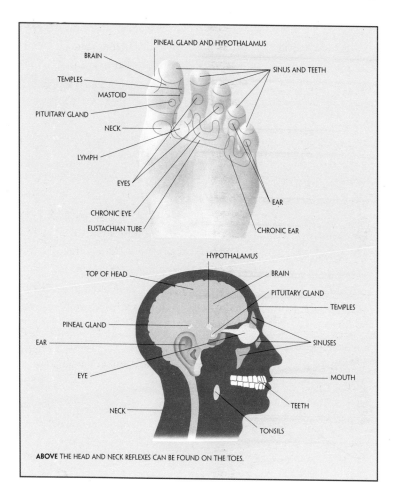

PINEAL GLAND AND HYPOTHALAMUS

BRAIN

TEMPLES

SINUS AND TEETH

MASTOID

PITUITARY GLAND

NECK

LYMPH

EYES

EAR

CHRONIC EYE

EUSTACHIAN TUBE

CHRONIC EAR

HYPOTHALAMUS

TOP OF HEAD

BRAIN

PITUITARY GLAND

TEMPLES

PINEAL GLAND

EAR

SINUSES

EYE

MOUTH

TEETH

NECK

TONSILS

ABOVE THE HEAD AND NECK REFLEXES CAN BE FOUND ON THE TOES.

65

THE PITUITARY GLAND

The pituitary gland, which is about the size and shape of a cherry, is attached to the base of the brain. Also known also as the 'master gland', the pituitary is considered the most important gland in the body as it controls the functions of all the endocrine glands. Numerous hormones are produced by the pituitary gland – these hormones influence growth, sexual development, metabolism, pregnancy, mineral and sugar contents of the blood, fluid retention and energy levels.

The reflex point is found on both feet where the whorl of the toe print converges into a central point. It is usually situated on the inner side of the toe and often requires a little searching. More often than not, this reflex is found to be off-centre. Since the hormonal system is extremely sensitive, this reflex is usually very tender.

THE HYPOTHALAMUS
A number of bodily activities are controlled by this part of the brain. It regulates the autonomic nervous system and controls emotional reactions, appetite, body temperature and sleep.

The hypothalamus reflex areas are found on both feet on the outer side and top of the big toe – the same reflex point as the pineal gland.

THE PINEAL GLAND
The pineal gland is a small gland situated within the hypothalamus section of the brain. Its functions are not completely understood, but it is known to stimulate the cells in the skin to produce the black pigment melanin. It is thought to play a part in mood and daily rhythms, and is sometimes referred to as the psychic 'third eye'.

The reflexes are on both feet on the outer tip of the big toes – the same as the hypothalamus reflex.

THE TEETH
The reflexes to the teeth are exactly distributed over the ten toes: incisors (1) on the big toe; incisors and canine teeth (2, 3) on the second toe; premolars (4, 5) on the third toe; molars (6, 7) on the fourth toe; wisdom teeth (8) on the fifth toe.

These reflexes are in the same position as the sinus reflexes.

THE EYES
The eyes are important sensory organs – the organs of sight. The retina receives impressions of images via the pupils and the lens. The optic nerve conveys the impressions from the receptors in the eye to the visual area of the cerebral cortex where they are interpreted.

These reflexes are on both feet on the cushions of the second and third toes and may extend slightly down the toes. Reflexes for chronic eye conditions are on the 'shelf' at the base of these two toes.

THE EARS

The ear is the organ of hearing. It is a highly complex system of cavities, bones and membranes, constructed in such a way that sound waves in the atmosphere are caught up and transmitted to the hearing centre in the temporal lobe of the cerebral cortex. The ear also plays a part in maintaining balance.

The reflexes are situated on both feet on the cushions of the fourth and fifth toes and may extend slightly down the toes. The reflexes for the eustachian tubes extend from the inner side of the big toe along the base of the second and third toes to the fourth toe. Reflexes for chronic ear conditions are found on the 'shelf' at the base of these two toes – the same section as the eustachian tubes. The mastoid – the part of the skull behind the ear that contains the air spaces that communicate with the ear – can also be treated on these reflexes.

67

THE TONSILS

These are paired organs composed of lymphatic tissue. They help to destroy micro-organisms in this area. These reflexes are found on both feet – on the top of the foot at the base of the big toe near the web between the big and second toes.

THE LYMPH SYSTEM

The lymphatic system forms a subsidiary or secondary circulatory system. It is a network of lymphatic vessels situated throughout the body that acts to drain tissue fluid surrounding the cells in the body. Lymph nodes filter the lymph to prevent infection passing into the blood stream and add lymphocytes, which are important for the formation of antibodies and immunological reactions. The main sites of the lymph nodes are in the neck, armpit, thorax, abdomen, groin, pelvis and behind the knee.

On the front of the foot, the webs between the toes are the reflexes for the drainage of the lymphatics in the neck/chest region of the body. Lymph reflexes for the groin area are tied in with the reproductive system and are found in the same area as the reflexes for the fallopian tubes and vas deferens (this will be described later in this chapter, *see* pp.81–82). These reflexes run across the top of the foot from the inner ankle bone to the outer ankle bone and incorporate the six main meridians.

Congestions in the groin can be traced to a specific meridian and its organ depending on where lumps are situated – proving the significance of the meridians.

THE THORACIC AREA – THE BALL OF THE FOOT

This section of the foot corresponds to the thoracic area in the body, from the shoulder girdle to the diaphragm. Several vital reflexes can be found here – the heart, lungs, oesophagus, trachea, bronchi, thyroid and thymus glands, diaphragm and solar plexus.

THE LUNGS

The lungs are cone-shaped, spongy organs in the thorax that lie on either side of the heart. It is here that the process of respiration takes place – the exchange of oxygen for carbon dioxide. The main air passage of the respiratory system found in the thorax is the trachea (also known as the windpipe), which divides into the bronchi to enter the left and right lungs.

The lung reflexes are found on the soles of both feet from the second toe (stomach meridian) to just past the fourth toe (gall bladder meridian). Reflexes of the trachea and bronchi are found below the big toe and second toes (stomach and liver meridians) connected to the lung reflex. These same reflexes are also found in similar positions on the tops of the feet.

THE BALL OF THE FOOT REFLEXES

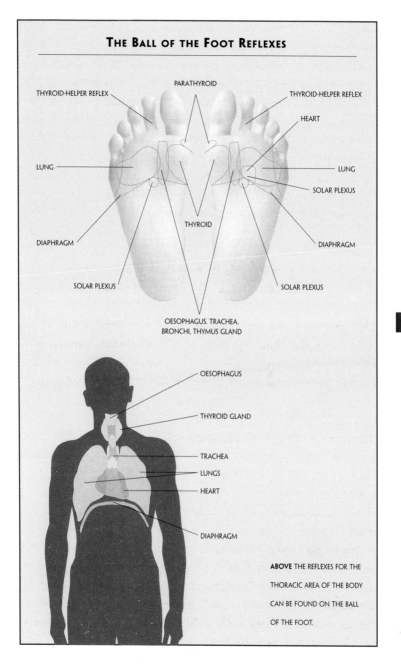

PARATHYROID

THYROID-HELPER REFLEX

THYROID-HELPER REFLEX

HEART

LUNG

LUNG

SOLAR PLEXUS

DIAPHRAGM

THYROID

DIAPHRAGM

SOLAR PLEXUS

SOLAR PLEXUS

OESOPHAGUS, TRACHEA, BRONCHI, THYMUS GLAND

69

OESOPHAGUS

THYROID GLAND

TRACHEA

LUNGS

HEART

DIAPHRAGM

ABOVE THE REFLEXES FOR THE
THORACIC AREA OF THE BODY
CAN BE FOUND ON THE BALL
OF THE FOOT.

THE HEART

The heart is a hollow, cone-shaped, muscular organ that lies in the chest on the left side of the body in a space between the lungs. It acts as a pump, circulating blood throughout the body. Good functioning of the heart is essential to allow good blood circulation throughout the body, which is necessary for efficient transport of gases, foods and waste products. The chest area also contains other major vessels leading to and from the heart – the vena cavae, aorta and other arteries and veins.

The reflex to the heart is situated on the sole of the left foot only – on the kidney meridian above the diaphragm level.

THE THYMUS GLAND, OESOPHAGUS, TRACHEA AND BRONCHI

The thymus gland is situated in the thoracic cavity. It is quite large in childhood, reaches maximum size at 10–12 years, then slowly regresses and has almost disappeared in adult life. It is involved in the immune system. The only known function of the thymus gland is the formation of lymphocytes.

The oesophagus is the gullet – a muscular tube passing from the pharynx down through the chest, and joining the stomach below the diaphragm. Food and fluid are propelled through the oesophagus by peristalsis (a wave-like contraction).

The trachea is the windpipe. It passes down from the larynx into the throat, where it divides into two main bronchi.

The bronchi are the two main divisions of the trachea, which enter the lungs.

All these reflexes can be found on both feet in the same area – that is, on the soles of the feet, in a vertical line between the first and second toes.

THE THYROID GLAND

The thyroid gland is located in the neck. It controls the rate of metabolism, which is necessary for normal mental and physical development, and also maintains the correct amount of calcium in the blood.

This reflex is situated on both feet at the base of the big toe, down around the ball and into the groove below the bone. The most important part is the section along the bone. There is also a 'helper' reflex on the second toe – the stomach meridian.

THE PARATHYROID GLANDS

These are four small glands situated around the thyroid gland. Their main function is to maintain the correct amount of calcium and phosphorus in the blood and bones.

The reflex is situated on both feet at the base of the big toe on the outer side.

THE DIAPHRAGM

The diaphragm, one of the muscles of respiration, is a large, dome-shaped wall that separates the thorax from the abdomen. It is the most important muscle for breathing.

This reflex is situated on the soles of both feet, and extends across all six meridians at the base of the ball of the foot separating the ball from the arch.

71

THE SOLAR PLEXUS

The solar plexus is a network of sympathetic nerve ganglia in the abdomen and is the nerve supply to the abdominal organs below the diaphragm. It is sometimes referred to as the 'abdominal brain' or the 'nerve switchboard' and is situated behind the stomach and in front of the diaphragm.

The reflex is at the same level as the reflex to the diaphragm located at a specific point in the centre of the diaphragm reflex. This point is visible on the foot as the apex of the arch that runs across the base of the ball of the foot. This reflex is most useful for inducing a relaxed state. It can relieve stress and nervousness, aid deep regular breathing and restore calm.

THE ABDOMINAL AREA – THE ARCH OF THE FOOT

The arch of the foot is clearly visible on the sole – the raised area that extends from the base of the ball to the start of the heel. It is divided into two parts – the upper part corresponds to the section of the body from the diaphragm to the waistline and the lower part corresponds to the section of the body from the waistline to the pelvic area.

Reflexes above the waistline – liver, gall bladder, stomach, pancreas, duodenum, spleen, adrenals and kidneys.

Reflexes below the waistline – small intestine, ileo-caecal valve, appendix, large intestine, adrenals, kidneys, ureters, bladder.

THE LIVER

The liver is the largest and most complex organ in the body. It has many functions including processing nutrients from the blood, storing fats, sugars and proteins, detoxifying the blood and manufacturing bile for fat digestion, storing sugars in the form of glycogen (to be used when the body needs an increased supply of energy) and the storage and metabolism of fats and proteins.

This reflex is found on the sole of the right foot only, below the diaphragm level, extending from the pancreas meridian on the inside of the foot to below the little toe. It ends just above the waistline.

THE GALL BLADDER

This is a small, muscular, pear-shaped sac attached to the under-surface of the liver. Its function is to excrete bile for food digestion.

The gall bladder reflex is on the sole of the right foot only, embedded within the liver reflex beneath and between the third and fourth toes.

THE STOMACH

The stomach is a large muscular bag that lies below the diaphragm mainly to the left side of the body. Food passes from the mouth down

THE ARCH REFLEXES

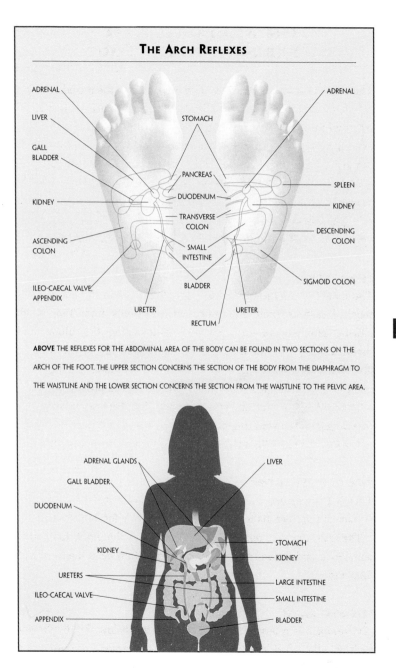

ADRENAL

LIVER

GALL
BLADDER

KIDNEY

ASCENDING
COLON

ILEO-CAECAL VALVE,
APPENDIX

STOMACH

PANCREAS

DUODENUM

TRANSVERSE
COLON

SMALL
INTESTINE

BLADDER

URETER

RECTUM

URETER

ADRENAL

SPLEEN

KIDNEY

DESCENDING
COLON

SIGMOID COLON

ABOVE THE REFLEXES FOR THE ABDOMINAL AREA OF THE BODY CAN BE FOUND IN TWO SECTIONS ON THE ARCH OF THE FOOT. THE UPPER SECTION CONCERNS THE SECTION OF THE BODY FROM THE DIAPHRAGM TO THE WAISTLINE AND THE LOWER SECTION CONCERNS THE SECTION FROM THE WAISTLINE TO THE PELVIC AREA.

73

ADRENAL GLANDS

GALL BLADDER

DUODENUM

KIDNEY

URETERS

ILEO-CAECAL VALVE

APPENDIX

LIVER

STOMACH

KIDNEY

LARGE INTESTINE

SMALL INTESTINE

BLADDER

the oesophagus into the stomach where it is churned up and mixed with gastric juices and enzymes to start the digestive process.

The reflexes are found on the soles of both feet – extending from the big toe to the second toe on the right foot and the big toe to the outer edge of the fourth toe on the left foot. Horizontally they are situated just below the diaphragm level.

THE PANCREAS

The pancreas is a large glandular structure in the abdomen. It is both an endocrine and exocrine gland secreting insulin and digestive juices. The pancreas is probably best known for its function as an endocrine gland and for the production of the two hormones insulin and glucagon, which both help to regulate the amount of sugars in the blood.

The reflexes are situated on the soles of both feet – more on the left foot than the right foot – below the stomach and above the waistline. On the right foot it extends into just below the big toe, and on the left foot as far as the fourth toe.

THE DUODENUM

This is the first, C-shaped part of the small intestine, about 20–25cm long. It extends from the pyloric sphincter of the stomach to the jejunum. Pancreatic and common bile ducts open into the duodenum, releasing secretions that are responsible for the breakdown of food in the body.

The reflexes are on the soles of both feet, immediately below the pancreas, touching the waistline and extending inwards to the second toe.

THE SPLEEN

The spleen is a large, very vascular, gland-like but ductless organ found on the left side of the body behind the stomach. It plays an important part in the immune system, and is part of the lymphatic system. It contains lymphatic tissue, which manufactures the white blood cells, breaks down old red blood corpuscles and filters the lymph of toxins.

The spleen reflex is found on the outer side of the left foot (opposite the liver reflex on the right foot), beneath the fourth toe (gall bladder meridian), just below the diaphragm line in line with the stomach reflex.

THE KIDNEYS

The kidneys are part of the main excretory system of the body – the urinary system – which collectively refers to the kidneys, ureter tubes, urethra and bladder. They are two bean-shaped organs that filter toxins from the blood, produce urine and regulate the retention of important minerals and water.

The reflexes are found on the soles of both feet positioned just above the waistline on the kidney and stomach meridians, just below the stomach reflex. The right kidney is positioned slightly lower than the left kidney.

75

THE ADRENAL GLANDS

These are two triangular endocrine glands situated on the upper tip of each kidney. As part of the endocrine system they perform numerous vital functions. The adrenal glands are divided into two distinct regions, the cortex and medulla. The adrenal cortex produces steroid hormones that regulate carbohydrate metabolism and have anti-allergic and anti-inflammatory properties. The cortex also produces hormones that control the reabsorption of sodium and water in the kidneys, as well as the secretion of potassium and the sex hormones testosterone and oestrogen.

The adrenal medulla produces adrenaline and noradrenaline that work in conjunction with the sympathetic nervous system. The output of adrenaline is increased at times of anxiety and stress and is responsible for organ changes in the 'fight-or-flight' situation.

The reflexes are situated on the soles of both feet on top of the kidney reflexes.

THE SMALL INTESTINE

This is a muscular tube about 6–7m in length. It is the main area of the digestive tract where absorption takes place. It leads from the pyloric sphincter of the stomach to the caecum of the large intestine and lies in a coiled position in the abdominal cavity surrounded by the large intestine. The small intestine is divided into three sections – the duodenum, jejunum and the ileum.

The reflex is situated on the soles of both feet, under the large intestine reflex just below the waistline to the end of the arch extending across to below the fourth toe.

THE ILEO-CAECAL VALVE

This valve is situated where the small intestine and large intestine join; it therefore controls the passage of contents of the small intestine through to the large intestine. It prevents backflow of faecal matter from the large intestine and controls mucus secretions.

The reflex is found on the sole of the right foot below and between the third and fourth toes just above the level of the pelvic floor.

THE APPENDIX

The appendix is a worm-like tube about 9–10cm in length with a blind end projecting downwards from the caecum of the large intestine in the lower right part of the abdominal cavity. Located directly below the ileo-caecal valve, it helps lubricate the large intestine, is rich in lymphoid tissue and secretes antibodies.

The reflex is situated only on the sole of the right foot, in the same area as the ileo-caecal valve.

THE LARGE INTESTINE

This is a tube about 1.5m in length. It starts on the right side of the body at the caecum (ileo-caecal valve) and goes up the right side to below the liver where it bends to the left (hepatic flexure) and passes across the abdomen as the transverse colon. At the left side of the abdomen, it bends down below the spleen (splenic flexure) to become the descending colon, which passes down the left side of the abdomen. It then turns towards the midline and takes the shape of a double S-shaped bend known as the sigmoid flexure. This leads into the rectum, which in turn leads to the anus.

When food residue reaches the large intestine it is in fluid form. The function of the large intestine is to remove some of the water and salts by absorption and to convert the waste matter into faeces ready for excretion.

The reflexes are found on the soles of both feet. On the right foot, the reflexes begin just below the reflex for the ileo-caecal valve and extends upwards (ascending colon), then turns just below the liver reflex to become the transverse colon, which extends across the entire foot. It continues across to the left foot and turns just below the spleen reflex to become the descending colon. Just above the pelvic floor it turns again into the sigmoid colon, which ends at the reflex of the rectum/anus.

77

THE URETERS

Ureter tubes are muscular tubes about 30cm in length that connect the kidneys and bladder and function as a passageway for urine. There are two tubes, one from each kidney, which pass downwards through the abdomen into the pelvis where they enter the bladder.

The reflexes are situated on the soles of both feet linking the kidney reflexes to the bladder reflexes, which are situated on the inner side of the instep. The ureter reflex can often be seen as distinct lines running across the arch.

THE BLADDER

The bladder is an elastic muscular sac situated in the centre of the pelvis. Urine passes from the kidneys down the ureters and is stored in the bladder until it is excreted via the urethra.

The reflexes are found on both feet on the side of the foot below the inner ankle bone on the heel line. This reflex is often clearly visible as a puffy area.

THE PELVIC AREA – THE HEEL OF THE FOOT

Although few organs are represented here, this area is of vital importance as all six main meridians traverse the pelvic section of the heel. As a result, many congestions found here can be traced to meridians and their organs.

THE SCIATIC NERVE

This is the largest nerve in the body. It arises from the sacral plexus of nerves formed by the lower lumbar and upper sacral spinal nerves. It runs from the buttocks down the back of the thigh and divides just above the knee into two main branches that supply the lower leg.

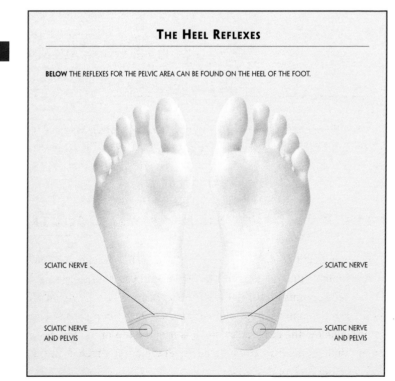

THE HEEL REFLEXES

BELOW THE REFLEXES FOR THE PELVIC AREA CAN BE FOUND ON THE HEEL OF THE FOOT.

SCIATIC NERVE

SCIATIC NERVE

SCIATIC NERVE AND PELVIS

SCIATIC NERVE AND PELVIS

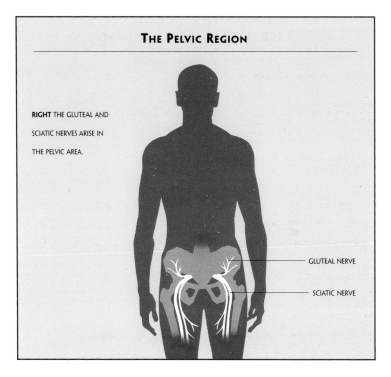

THE PELVIC REGION

RIGHT THE GLUTEAL AND SCIATIC NERVES ARISE IN THE PELVIC AREA.

GLUTEAL NERVE

SCIATIC NERVE

The sciatic nerve and reflex are found on the soles of both feet – in a band about a third of the way down the pad of the heel extending right across the foot.

THE REPRODUCTIVE AREA – THE ANKLE

The outer ankle contains the ovaries/testes reflexes, and the inner ankle contains the uterus, prostate, vagina and penis reflexes.

The reflex points for the fallopian tubes, lymph drainage area in the groin, vas deferens and seminal vesicles are found in a narrow band running below the outer ankle bone across the top of the foot to the inner ankle bone. The kidney/bladder meridian is situated on both sides up the back of the ankle.

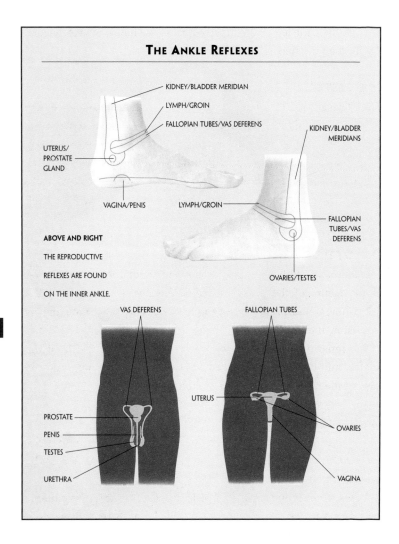

THE ANKLE REFLEXES

KIDNEY/BLADDER MERIDIAN

LYMPH/GROIN

FALLOPIAN TUBES/VAS DEFERENS

KIDNEY/BLADDER MERIDIANS

UTERUS/ PROSTATE GLAND

VAGINA/PENIS

LYMPH/GROIN

FALLOPIAN TUBES/VAS DEFERENS

ABOVE AND RIGHT

THE REPRODUCTIVE

REFLEXES ARE FOUND

ON THE INNER ANKLE.

OVARIES/TESTES

VAS DEFERENS

FALLOPIAN TUBES

UTERUS

PROSTATE

PENIS

TESTES

URETHRA

OVARIES

VAGINA

THE OVARIES

These are the female sex glands. There are two ovaries – one on each side of the uterus. These are part of the female reproductive system and produce ova as well as the hormones oestrogen and progesterone.

The reflexes are found on both feet on the outer side, midway between the ankle bone and the back of the heel – the right ovary on the right foot, the left ovary on the left foot. The helper area is the heel due to the presence of the meridians.

THE TESTES

The testes are the male reproductive glands that produce spermatozoa and the male hormone testosterone. There are two testes suspended outside the body in the scrotum – a sack of thin, dark-coloured skin that lies behind the penis.

The reflexes are found on males in the same area as the ovaries in females, that is, midway between the outer ankle bone and the heel. The helper area is the heel.

THE UTERUS

The uterus is a hollow, pear-shaped organ about 10cm long situated in the centre of the pelvic cavity in females. Its function is the nourishment and protection of the foetus during pregnancy and its expulsion at term.

The reflex points are located on both feet on the inside of the ankles, midway on a diagonal line between the ankle bone and the back of the heel. The helper area is the heel.

THE PROSTATE GLAND

This gland lies at the base of the male bladder and surrounds the urethra. It produces the thin lubricating fluid that forms part of the semen, which aids the transportation of sperm cells.

Reflexes are found on both feet in the same place as the uterus reflex on females – midway in a diagonal line between the inner ankle bone and the heel. Again, the heel is the helper area.

THE FALLOPIAN TUBES

In females, these two tubes, about 10–14cm in length, connect the ovaries with the cavity of the uterus. Their function is to conduct the ova, which is expelled from the ovaries during ovulation, down the tube to the uterus.

The reflexes are found on both feet. They run across the top of the foot linking the reflex of the uterus to the reflex of the ovaries. This area is usually massaged in conjunction with the reflexes of the ovaries and uterus.

THE SEMINAL VESICLES/VAS DEFERENS

The seminal vesicles lie next to the prostate and store semen. The vas deferens are a pair of excretory ducts that convey semen from the testes through the prostate and into the urethra.

The reflexes are located in the same area as the fallopian tubes in females – across the top of the foot from one ankle bone to the other, linking the prostate and testes reflexes.

THE SPINE - THE INNER FOOT

The inside of each foot is naturally curved to correspond to the spine.

THE SPINE

The spine, also known as the backbone or vertebral column, is the central support of the body. It carries the weight of the body and is an important axis of movement. The spine is made up of 33 vertebrae. The structure of the bones is arranged in such a way as to give the spine four curves. The spine is divided into four sections from top to bottom: seven cervical vertebrae (including the first two, axis and atlas) = the neck; 12 thoracic vertebrae = the back; five lumbar vertebrae = the loin; five sacral vertebrae = the pelvis; four/five coccycal vertebrae = the tail. The vertebrae of the sacrum and coccyx are fused to form two immobile bones. Vertebrae are joined by discs of cartilage and are held in place by ligaments.

The spinal column encloses the spinal cord, the central channel of the nervous system, which is a continuation of the brain stem. It carries the nerves from the brain to all parts of the body. A spinal nerve is associated with each vertebra. These nerves arise from the

THE INNER FOOT REFLEXES

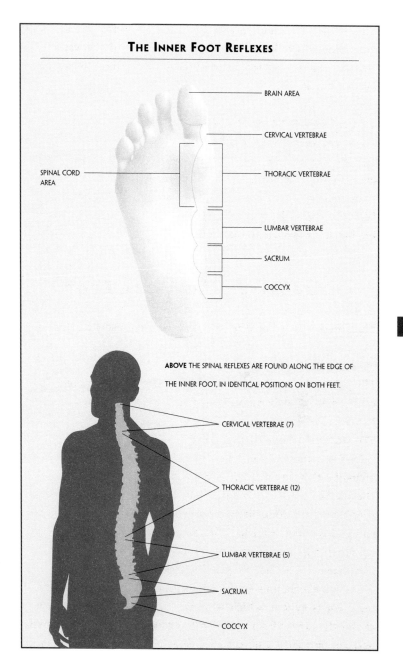

BRAIN AREA

CERVICAL VERTEBRAE

SPINAL CORD AREA

THORACIC VERTEBRAE

LUMBAR VERTEBRAE

SACRUM

COCCYX

ABOVE THE SPINAL REFLEXES ARE FOUND ALONG THE EDGE OF THE INNER FOOT, IN IDENTICAL POSITIONS ON BOTH FEET.

CERVICAL VERTEBRAE (7)

THORACIC VERTEBRAE (12)

LUMBAR VERTEBRAE (5)

SACRUM

COCCYX

83

spinal cord and affect the level of the body at which they arise – that is, the thoracic nerves affect the thorax, and the lumbar nerves the lower abdomen and legs.

The reflex zones run along the inner side of both feet – half the spine represented on each foot. The cervical vertebrae reflex runs from the base of the big toe nail to the base of the toe (between the first and second joints of the big toe). The thoracic reflex runs along the ball of the foot below the big toe (shoulder to waistline), the arch from the waistline to pelvic line corresponds to the lumbar region and the heel line to the base of the heel to the sacrum/coccyx.

THE OUTER FOOT – THE OUTER BODY

The outer edge of the foot corresponds to the outer part of the body – the joints, ligaments and surrounding muscles. From the base of the toe to the diaphragm line = shoulder and upper arm; diaphragm line to waistline = elbow, forearm, wrist and hand; waistline to end of heel = leg, knee and hip.

THE KNEE
The knee joint joins the upper and lower leg.

Reflexes are found on both feet on the outer side, just below the bony projection of the fifth metatarsal, which is usually quite prominent on the side of the foot. Again, remember that the six meridians run through the knee, so by pinpointing the exact location of the knee pain, one can relate it to a specific meridian and locate the problematic organ.

THE HIP
The hip joint is where the thigh bone (femur) meets the pelvis.

The reflex is found on both feet extending towards the toe in front of the knee reflex. It covers a half moon shape, moving out from the line along the side of the foot and up in line with one

THE OUTER FOOT REFLEXES

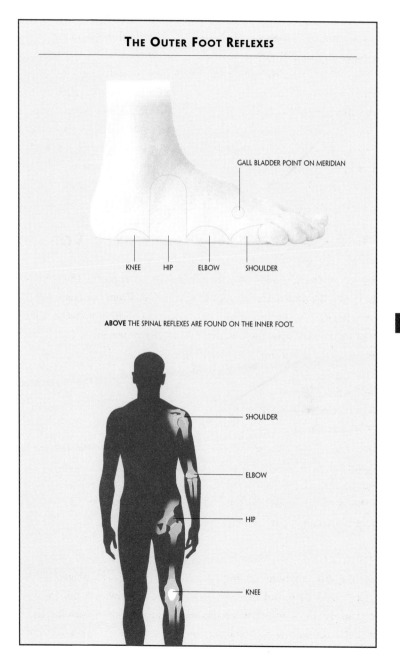

GALL BLADDER POINT ON MERIDIAN

KNEE   HIP   ELBOW   SHOULDER

ABOVE THE SPINAL REFLEXES ARE FOUND ON THE INNER FOOT.

SHOULDER

ELBOW

HIP

KNEE

fourth toe and the gall bladder meridian. Some hip problems may be gall bladder related, as the gall bladder meridian passes directly through the hip.

THE ELBOW AND SHOULDER

The elbow is the joint between the upper arm and the forearm.

It is formed by the humerus above, and the radius and ulna below. The shoulder joint is where the bone of the upper arm (humerus) meets the shoulder blade (scapula).

The reflexes to the elbow are situated on both feet on the outer side along the arch and the ball. The shoulder and the surrounding muscles are found on both feet at the base of the fifth toe covering the sole, outer side and top.

THE TOP OF THE FOOT – THE BREAST AREA AND CIRCULATION POINTS

Reflexes found on the top of the foot include the circulation and breast. Most of the reflexes represented on the soles are also found on the tops of the feet in the meridians.

THE BREAST

It is important to look at the meridians here. If there are breast problems, note exactly where these are situated so as to identify the meridian that runs through the affected section of the breast and thereby the problem organ.

SPECIAL CIRCULATION POINTS

These points are to stimulate the heart, circulation and body temperature. These are found on the top and soles of both feet at the web between the second and third toes. As these are points on the stomach meridian, they have an effect on the thyroid, which in turn affects body temperature, heart and circulation.

THE TOP OF FOOT REFLEXES

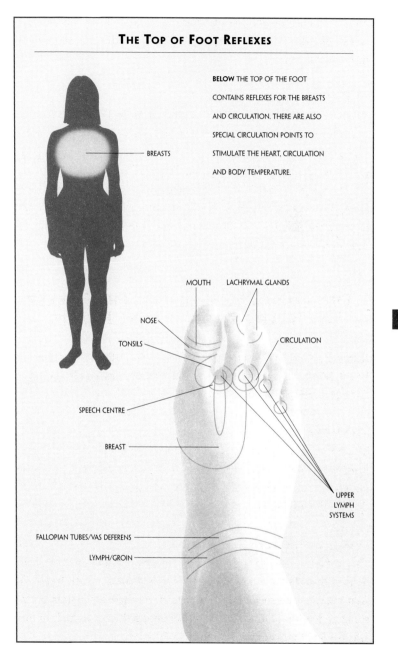

BELOW THE TOP OF THE FOOT CONTAINS REFLEXES FOR THE BREASTS AND CIRCULATION. THERE ARE ALSO SPECIAL CIRCULATION POINTS TO STIMULATE THE HEART, CIRCULATION AND BODY TEMPERATURE.

BREASTS

MOUTH

LACHRYMAL GLANDS

NOSE

CIRCULATION

TONSILS

SPEECH CENTRE

BREAST

UPPER LYMPH SYSTEMS

FALLOPIAN TUBES/VAS DEFERENS

LYMPH/GROIN

READING THE FEET

CHAPTER FIVE

It is estimated that approximately 80 per cent of adults will develop foot disorders, even though most people are born with healthy feet. There is an overriding tendency to blame foot problems and deformities such as corns, callouses and bunions on ill-fitting shoes. These undoubtedly form part of the problem, but only a part. Problem areas on the feet relate to problem areas within the body. Which is the cause and which is the effect is debatable. It is a 'chicken or egg' situation. Congestions along a meridian will disrupt the body's equilibrium – be they internal or external. If the problem is internal, the reflex area and the relevant meridian will be particularly sensitive to excess pressure and friction and more susceptible to the formations of corns and callouses. However, these external problems can also cause congestions along the meridians in the same way as internal congestions. If these are not dealt with, then they can have an adverse effect on body parts along the whole meridian, thus creating an imbalance throughout the body.

With our knowledge of reflexes and meridians, we can now look at these problems in a new light and unravel the tales they have to tell about the state of the body as a whole. The areas where the problems show themselves are particularly significant when integrating the concept of meridians.

BUNIONS

A bunion is a prominence of the head of the metatarsal bone at its junction with the big toe. It is caused by inflammation and swelling of the bursa (bursitis) at that joint. The bursa is a pocket of fluid enclosed in fibrous tissue that surrounds the joints and serves to protect them from friction. The metatarsal joint becomes enlarged with a bunion and is therefore subject to pressure and friction from shoes, which further aggravate the problem and damage the skin.

As the bunion develops, the big toe moves sideways, constricting and displacing the other toes – particularly the second toe, which is forced out of alignment into a position on top of the big toe. This is known as a hammertoe and it may, in time, become permanently bent. Its position above the other toes makes it prone to corns and callouses on the top of the toe due mainly to pressure from shoes.

The constriction of the toes can also affect the little toe – forcing it towards the middle of the foot and causing a 'bunionette' on the outer side at the base of the little toe.

WHAT MERIDIANS REVEAL ABOUT BUNIONS

Two important meridians are found on the big toe – the spleen/pancreas meridian on the outer side and the liver meridian on the inner side towards the second toe. Bunions are situated on the pancreas meridian and the thyroid reflex. The internal branch of the spleen/pancreas meridian runs through the thyroid, further indicating their close relationship. Most people with bunions also have problems along the spleen/pancreas meridian or pancreatic disorders. For example, problems related to sugar metabolism such as a sweet tooth, cravings for stimulants such as tea, coffee, cigarettes and alcohol and constant hunger. They may suffer from depression due to the fact that the thyroid is affected. Many people who have had bunions removed or repaired at an early age often develop thyroid problems in later life. Or vice versa – people with thyroid

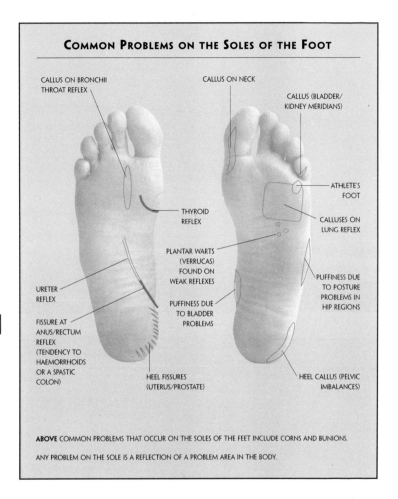

COMMON PROBLEMS ON THE SOLES OF THE FOOT

CALLUS ON BRONCHII THROAT REFLEX

CALLUS ON NECK

CALLUS (BLADDER/ KIDNEY MERIDIANS)

THYROID REFLEX

ATHLETE'S FOOT

CALLUSES ON LUNG REFLEX

PLANTAR WARTS (VERRUCAS) FOUND ON WEAK REFLEXES

URETER REFLEX

PUFFINESS DUE TO BLADDER PROBLEMS

PUFFINESS DUE TO POSTURE PROBLEMS IN HIP REGIONS

FISSURE AT ANUS/RECTUM REFLEX (TENDENCY TO HAEMORRHOIDS OR A SPASTIC COLON)

HEEL FISSURES (UTERUS/PROSTATE)

HEEL CALLUS (PELVIC IMBALANCES)

ABOVE COMMON PROBLEMS THAT OCCUR ON THE SOLES OF THE FEET INCLUDE CORNS AND BUNIONS.

ANY PROBLEM ON THE SOLE IS A REFLECTION OF A PROBLEM AREA IN THE BODY.

problems often develop bunions. This is because the underlying causes of the symptom – the pancreas and thyroid imbalances – have not been corrected.

Once a bunion has developed in an adult foot it cannot be realigned or straightened without surgery. No exercise or manipulation will push it back. However, by understanding the connection with the meridians, we can understand the cause of the problem – a pancreas imbalance – and set about rectifying that. This

PROBLEMS ON THE TOP OF THE FOOT

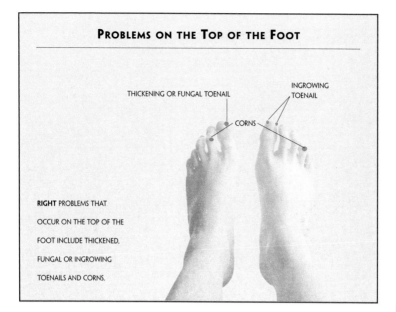

THICKENING OR FUNGAL TOENAIL

INGROWING TOENAIL

CORNS

RIGHT PROBLEMS THAT OCCUR ON THE TOP OF THE FOOT INCLUDE THICKENED, FUNGAL OR INGROWING TOENAILS AND CORNS.

HAMMERTOE

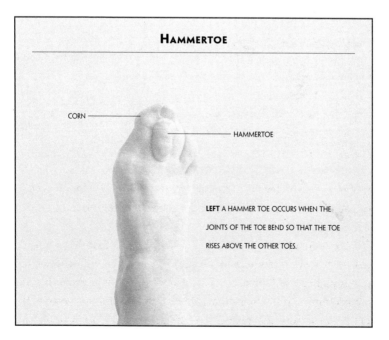

CORN

HAMMERTOE

LEFT A HAMMER TOE OCCURS WHEN THE JOINTS OF THE TOE BEND SO THAT THE TOE RISES ABOVE THE OTHER TOES.

problem is most effectively rectified by a change of diet. Pain caused by bunions can be significantly alleviated with reflexology treatments and a change of diet.

CORNS AND CALLOUSES

Corns usually develop on the joints of the toes that, due to their relative prominence, are particularly sensitive to pressure from shoes. At the focal point of this pressure, the skin hardens and thickens. A corn – basically a concentrated area of hard skin – forms in the middle of the area of thickening where the pressure is greatest. Corns also develop on the soles of the feet in areas of excessive pressure. The stabbing pain that is often characteristic of corns is caused by the hard skin exerting secondary pressure onto the sensitive tissue and nerve endings beneath it.

Repeated pressure and friction on the skin will cause it to thicken as a means of protection. Foot callouses are quite common since the skin on the feet is subject to a great deal of pressure – particularly from ill-fitting shoes. If this thickening is aggravated by consistent pressure, the build-up of skin will lead to pain and discomfort. Callouses are especially visible on the tops of the toes and soles of the feet. They are easily removed by a chiropodist but will recur if the reason for their formation is not dealt with.

MERIDIANS AND CORNS AND CALLOUSES

Corns and callouses usually develop on the tops of the toes. It is important to note exactly where these appear and establish on which meridian they manifest and in turn which organs are out of balance. For example, the stomach meridian runs along the second and third toes, and problems here indicate congestions along the stomach meridian. Symptoms such as acidity, gastritis, ulcers, appendix and tonsil trouble, sinus, skin problems and breast problems are often found in people with problems on the second and third toes.

The second and third toes are also often longer than the first toe. This can indicate a genetic weakness in the stomach, often inherited, but can also be due to dietary deficiencies during the embryonic period. If the weakness is genetic, care should always be taken with diet – for example, avoiding excessively acid foods.

Some people have a long callous under the second toe. This relates to the bronchi/throat reflex area. If there is a deep groove in the skin, it could also relate to a weakness in the throat, and the person may have a tendency to suffer from throat, tonsil and bronchial problems. The stomach meridian traverses through the throat area – tonsils, thyroid and the throat itself. The stomach meridian is on top of the second toe while the throat and bronchial reflexes are on the soles between the first and second toes. Moving down, the meridian runs underneath the bone region – the thyroid. Many people have a groove or hard callous around the bone that, again, can be related to an imbalance in the thyroid region. This is often due to an imbalance in the spleen/pancreas and stomach meridians, as these two are very closely related. Hard skin over the lung reflex is also a common problem. This can indicate a weak chest. The stomach meridian also runs through the lung area and the gall bladder meridian enters the lung area from the side. As you can see, it is important to take careful note of where corns and callouses form and refer them to the meridians in order to understand the root cause of the problem.

ATHLETE'S FOOT

Athlete's foot is a fungal infection that usually manifests on the skin between the toes. This is the most common site of infection as the moist, warm conditions stimulate the fungus to multiply. The fungus thrives on keratin – a protein found in the outer layers of the skin. A major symptom of this condition is itching. If this itchiness is also accompanied by loose scaly skin surrounding patches of pink, exposed skin, then it is a sure sign of infection.

Occasionally a fissure – a split in the skin – may occur at the base of the toes. If this is deep, there could be a problem with bleeding. It could also be infected with bacteria and become inflamed if care is not taken. According to medical belief, athlete's foot is very easily transmitted to others, particularly where there is communal bathing.

MERIDIANS AND ATHLETE'S FOOT

Again, it is important to take note of exactly where on the foot the problem occurs. Athlete's foot will most often manifest in between the fourth and fifth toes – the bladder meridian – and can therefore be related to the bladder. If between the third and fourth toe, it is related to the gall bladder meridian.

TOENAIL PROBLEMS

Ingrowing toenails can be very painful and uncomfortable as anyone who suffers from this problem will know. Interestingly, those most often affected by this condition are young people in their teens and 20s. It usually occurs on the big toe when the side of the nail penetrates the skin of the nail groove and becomes embedded in the soft skin tissue. If the wound is hampered in its efforts to heal, it produces granulation tissue that accumulates on the side and top of the nail. This tissue bleeds very easily. Ingrowing toenails can be caused by cutting the nail too short or cutting down the sides of the nail. Thin brittle nails and moist skin will increase susceptibility to this problem.

An involuted toenail, if not correctly tended, can develop into an ingrowing toenail. This condition occurs when the normal curve of the toenail is so exaggerated that it produces pain down the side of the nail. The exaggerated curve can also encourage the development of corns and callouses on the sides of the nail, which will increase discomfort. It is difficult to cut this type of nail, but cutting down the sides must be avoided, as this will result in the new nail growth forcing its way through the soft skin at the side of the nail, causing an ingrowing toenail.

A toenail will thicken if the nail cell production centre is damaged. This can happen if the nail is persistently rubbed against a shoe over a prolonged period, or if the toenail has sustained injury in an accident. Unfortunately, this condition is irreversible. A further complication arises as the nail grows – the new growth curves – and is uncomfortable and unsightly. This curvature is known as a ram's-horn nail. Many elderly people are afflicted by this problem.

Fungal infection of the toenail often accompanies athlete's foot. The fungus penetrates the nail causing it to thicken. If the condition deteriorates, the colour and texture of the nail will also be affected, becoming darker and 'crumbly'.

MERIDIANS AND TOENAIL PROBLEMS

With all toenail troubles, it is important that meridians are taken into account. Take, for example, ingrowing toenails. This problem is often found in young people and situated on the big toe – the spleen/pancreas meridian mentioned earlier. These people usually have a diet high in sugar, junk food, alcohol, cigarettes – and many of their problems can be related to sugar metabolism or pancreatic disorders. They might also suffer from severe migraines or headaches. Remember that the big toe is also the head reflex. Over the years, I have seen many cases of clients suffering from headaches who also had ingrown toenails. Check the section on meridians, and note which meridians run through the area of the foot where the physical deformities and problems are found, in order to ascertain which organ is faulty and needs correcting.

PLANTAR DIGITAL NEURITIS

Neuritis is the inflammation of a nerve, with pain, tenderness and loss of function. This particular form of neuritis affects the toes, usually the fourth toe. The pain usually begins at the web between the third and fourth toes and shoots up into the fourth toe. The sensations experienced in the toe may vary from slight numbness to intense pain, depending on how severely the nerve is affected. The discomfort can be alleviated by massaging the toe. This problem usually occurs in women.

MERIDIANS AND PLANTAR DIGITAL NEURITIS

The gall bladder meridian is found on the fourth toe, where this problem is most common. Plantar digital neuritis is found in many women, and I have witnessed numerous cases where women have this problem around premenstrual time when they often crave chocolates, caffeine and other stimulants. The condition can therefore be related to overloading of the gall bladder meridian. Often symptoms will indicate other gall bladder related problems. This can also be associated with hip trouble – and can possibly be seen as a puffy area in line with the fourth toe close to the ankle. The gall bladder meridian runs through the hip region, and swelling here may indicate congestions along the gall bladder meridian.

96

FLAT FEET

Flat feet can be caused by numerous factors. They are generally inherited, but flat feet may also develop due to weakness in the joints or 'overloading' the feet, or they may be the result of a long illness. In childhood, this condition can occur if growth is too rapid, or if the child is malnourished or overweight. The weaker the foot, the greater the chance of this condition developing. Apart from causing an unattractive style of walking, flat feet can also affect the spine.

In flat feet, the arch of the foot is flattened and sinks. This causes over-stretching and weakness of both

ABOVE IN FLAT FEET, THE ARCH OF THE FOOT IS FLATTENED CAUSING THE SOLE TO LIE FLAT ON THE GROUND.

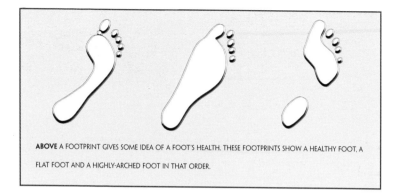

ABOVE A FOOTPRINT GIVES SOME IDEA OF A FOOT'S HEALTH. THESE FOOTPRINTS SHOW A HEALTHY FOOT, A FLAT FOOT AND A HIGHLY-ARCHED FOOT IN THAT ORDER.

muscles and tendons and places a strain on the bone structure. Another problem is that the nerves and blood vessels, which are usually protected from contact with the ground by the shape of the arch, are now subject to increased pressure and their condition will deteriorate affecting the reflexes in this area.

THE HIGHLY ARCHED FOOT

A highly arched foot is usually stiff, which limits movement and prevents efficient functioning of the foot. Due to the exaggerated height of the arch, the toes will not have correct contact with the ground when standing. The unnatural shape and position of the toes makes them susceptible to external pressures and therefore prone to corns and callouses. This condition may be inherited or could be the result of nerve and muscle imbalance. It is often seen in the neurological conditions poliomyelitis and spina bifida.

As a reflexologist, I would see the problem of flat feet as related to a rigid spine, indicating that the person is not very supple and who could also be prone to lower back problems. A highly curved arch or curved spine reflex also indicates a spinal problem, and this can cause problems with the upper part of the body – the lung area. If you press your fist against the lung reflex of the foot and gently press the foot back into a normal position, you will see the spinal reflex 'correcting' itself, and can therefore deduce that the client has a tendency to lower back problems, neck tension, congestions in the lung area and, as the toes are often also affected, problems along the meridians found in the toes.

THE HEEL

As the heel is subject to immense stress and bears a great deal of body weight, it has an extra protection of a thick layer of fatty tissue under the heel bone.

Heel callous is formed when areas of skin around the edge of the heel become thicker than usual to protect it from aggravating pressure and friction. It can develop into a painful condition if not dealt with.

A heel fissure develops when the skin on the edge of the heel splits. This is usually due to the fact that the skin is excessively dry and is being pinched by ill-fitting shoes. If the fissure is deep, pain and bleeding can occur.

REFLEXES/MERIDIANS AND HEEL PROBLEMS

The heel is the pelvic reflex, and problems here often indicate prostate problems in men and uterus problems in women. Many women have deep cracks in their heel just prior to a hysterectomy and these often heal naturally after the operation. Any other reproductive problems in men and women – infertility, heavy bleeding and discomfort – can be related to imbalances in the pelvic region. All six main meridians run through this area and organs and meridians can be stimulated by massage here.

ABOVE PRESSURE AND FRICTION MAY CAUSE THE HEEL TO DEVELOP A CALLOUS OR FISSURE.

TECHNIQUES

The body is reflected on the feet in a three-dimensional form. In the body, the organs overlap each other; therefore the reflex areas do the same on the feet. Many organs are minute and are not reflected on the charts, but all are worked on in the step-by-step treatment sequence. In the massage technique that I teach, treatment always includes both feet. The reflex areas of both left and right feet are alternately massaged from toes to heel. By contrast, many of the reflexology books available teach the 'thumb walking' technique and propose working one foot completely before moving on to the next. However, it is the prerogative of each individual practitioner to choose which technique works best for them as they all work equally well.

The most important aspect of the treatment procedure described in this chapter is that BOTH FEET ARE WORKED THROUGH ALTERNATELY FROM TOP TO TOE. This facilitates a natural flow in the procedure. One foot represents half a body, and as many organs are paired and found on both sides of the body, it would be wrong to complete one foot at a time. This would mean that only half the organ had been stimulated. The theory behind alternating feet is to stimulate each organ completely before moving on to the next. In this way, each body part is worked as a unit even though half is on the left foot and half on the right.

HOLDING THE FOOT

The first priority is to learn proper support or the pressure techniques will never be mastered correctly. The hands perform complementary functions throughout the treatment. While one hand presses, the other braces and supports or pushes the foot towards the pressure. To simplify things, the hand applying pressure will be referred to as the 'working hand' and the other hand the 'supporting hand'. Neither hand should ever be idle.

There is one main support technique. This is referred to as the standard support grip. Take the foot in the support hand, either from the inside or the outside – the web of the hand between the thumb and the index finger touching the side of the foot with the four fingers on top of the foot and the thumb on the sole. The support hand must always stay close to the working hand. Whichever grip you use on whatever reflex, always keep the foot bent slightly towards you and never in a tight grip with the toes bent backwards.

100

PRESSURE TECHNIQUES

THE ROTATING THUMB TECHNIQUE

This is the most important technique to master, as it is used to apply pressure to most of the reflexes throughout the treatment procedure. It is combined with finger techniques.

LEFT CORRECT SUPPORT IS VERY IMPORTANT IN REFLEXOLOGY.
THE MAIN TECHNIQUE USED FOR HOLDING THE FOOT IS THE
STANDARD SUPPORT GRIP.

Before working on the feet, exercise the 'rotating thumb' technique on the palm of your hand. It helps to visualize the object being worked on (hand or foot) as divided into small squares, all of which must be systematically stimulated. As you work, move from square to square, apply pressure and rotation to each square. The movement of the thumb from point to point must be small, moving along progressively, leaving no space between the points covered by the thumb tip.

For this exercise, place the four fingers of the working hand on the back of the hand to be worked on, keeping the thumb free to work on the palm. Bend the thumb from the first joint to between a 75 and 90 degree angle – the angle must ensure that the thumb nail does not dig into the flesh. This is the standard position of the 'rotating thumb'. The contact point is the tip of the thumb. Apply firm pressure with the tip of the thumb to the point to be worked on, and rotate the thumb, clockwise or anticlockwise. Keep the firm pressure constant and stay on the square. Two to three rotations are sufficient. Lift the thumb, move to the next point and repeat the procedure. The basic movement is press in, rotate, lift, move. The choice to increase the amount of pressure or number of rotations depends on the practitioner and patient.

Observe the movement of the thumb on the working hand. The most visible rotation must be at the second thumb joint – where the metacarpals of the hand join the phalanges of the thumb. Make sure you keep the thumb bent and the shoulders down to help with this technique. There should be very little strain on the arm muscles, elbows, neck and shoulders.

Furthermore, you will notice how much more pressure can be applied with the thumb in a bent position as opposed to a flat thumb. Ensure that the distance between the thumb and fist is sufficient to allow for easy rotation movements – approximately 2cm apart. By exercising the correct technique, the treatment procedure should not be at all strenuous for the practitioner. Practise this thumb rotating technique on your hand until you feel completely comfortable with it. Also ensure that you exercise the thumbs on both hands to enable you to work efficiently with either thumb, as it is important to be able to switch hands during the treatment sequence.

FINGER TECHNIQUES

1 Hands are placed on either side of the foot with the thumbs on the sole and four fingers on top. The index and third fingers are the working tools, the third finger usually placed on top of the index finger to create extra leverage. This is used on the fallopian tubes/vas deferens and lymphatic reflexes, which run from the outside ankle bone along the top of the foot at the ankle joint to the inside ankle bone. With the fingers, press in, rotate, lift and move as with the 'rotating thumb', moving point by point up both sides until the fingers meet at the centre on top of the foot.

2 This is used on the sides and tops of the toes. Place the index finger on one side and thumb on the other side of the toe to be worked on. 'Rub' the toe, moving the fingers gently back and forth in opposite directions.

3 Use both hands. Place the hands on either side of the foot, thumbs on the sole forming the support and four fingers on top.

The eight fingers are the working tools. Starting from the ankle joint, exert deep, smooth pressure with the fingers massaging down the foot towards the toes – slowly

ABOVE THIS FINGER TECHNIQUE IS USED ON THE FALLOPIAN TUBES/VAS DEFERENS REFLEXES.

and gently, but with firm pressure. Repeat this procedure a few times. Improvise a bit, but massage well. Also use a criss-cross movement with the thumbs on the sole of the foot. This is usually part of the winding down stage of the treatment that culminates in the solar plexus breathing technique. Cream or oil can be used at this stage to aid easy movement.

PINCH TECHNIQUE

The support hand cups the foot at the ankle, while the working hand locates the tendon at the back of the heel and moves up and down the tendon pinching this tendon gently between the thumb and the index finger.

This is used to stimulate the kidney and bladder meridian.

103

LEFT WITH THE PINCH TECHNIQUE THE WORKING HAND MOVES UP AND DOWN THE ACHILLES TENDON AT THE BACK OF THE HEEL.

KNEAD TECHNIQUE

This is a relatively easy technique, much like kneading bread. It is used mainly on the heel area, which is usually rather tough, and therefore needs more pressure for effective stimulation. Cup the ankle in the palm of the support hand, keeping the heel area free. Make a fist with the working hand, then use the knuckles of the second joint of the fingers to 'knead' the heel. This is used for working reflexes in the heel – the sciatic reflex and nerve and the reproductive reflexes.

These are the main basic finger and thumb techniques used in the treatment procedure. As one of the main benefits of reflexology is the relaxation aspect, it is important to become familiar with a few basic relaxation techniques.

LEFT KNEADING IS USED TO WORK ON AREAS THAT ARE THICK OR INSENSITIVE AND NEED EXTRA STIMULATION. THE HEEL IS ONE SUCH EXAMPLE.

RELAXATION TECHNIQUES

ACHILLES TENDON STRETCH

Cup the heel of one foot so that it rests in the palm of the hand. Grasp the top of the foot near the toes in the standard support grip. Pull the top of the foot towards you, allowing the heel to move backwards, then reverse the procedure, pulling the heel towards you and pushing the top of the foot backwards so that the bottom of the foot stretches out. Repeat this two or three times.

ABOVE THE ACHILLES TENDON STRETCH IS USED TO STRETCH THE BACK OF THE LEG AND RELEASE TENSION.

ANKLE ROTATION

Cup the back of the ankle of the right foot in the palm of the left (support) hand, with the thumb on the outside of the ankle and the fingers on the inside. Ensure a firm but not tight grasp. Working with the right hand from the inside of the foot, grasp the foot at the base of the big toe in the standard support grip. Hold the foot with equal pressure. Use the hand holding the ankle joint as a pivot, and rotate the foot with the right hand in 360 degree circles, first clockwise a few times, then anticlockwise. Work the other foot the same way alternating hands accordingly. Do not force the foot into exaggerated circles, manoeuvre it slowly and gently only as far as is comfortable for the client. This movement must be carried out smoothly and affects the entire area of the hip joint and tailbone, relaxes the anus and surrounding area and affects all the lower back muscles.

ABOVE THE ANKLE ROTATION CAN EASE MUSCULAR TENSION IN THE HIP JOINT AND TAILBONE AREA.

SIDE TO SIDE

This method of vigorously shaking the foot helps circulation, eases tenderness, and relaxes ankle and calf muscles. Place both palms on either side of the foot just above the ankles. Keep the hands as relaxed and loose as possible. Do not force the foot to rotate further than is comfortable for the patient.

Roll the foot from side to side by gently moving it back and forth between your hands, which move in opposite directions from each other. Move the hands gradually up the sides of the feet until the entire foot is worked. This is usually executed slowly to release tension, relax the edges of the ankle and calf and stimulate the whole foot.

LOOSEN ANKLES

Hook the base of both palms above the back sides of the heel so that the palms cover the ankle bones. The ankle joint serves as the pivot point. Move the hands rapidly backwards and forwards in opposite directions to each other, keeping the hands hooked beneath

ABOVE THE TECHNIQUE TO LOOSEN THE ANKLES SHOULD HELP ALL THE JOINTS IN THE BODY.

105

the ankle bones. The foot will shake from side to side when this movement is carried out properly.

THE SPINAL TWIST

Grasp the foot from the inside of the instep with both hands, fingers on top, thumbs on the sole – the web between the thumb and the index finger on the spinal reflex. The index fingers of each hand should be touching. When working the right foot, the right hand starting position will be at the ankle joint on the top of the foot and vice versa on

ABOVE THE SPINAL TWIST IS A RELAXING AND ENJOYABLE TECHNIQUE AND IS USED BY REFLEXOLOGISTS TO REDUCE TENSION.

the left foot. The hand close to the ankle will provide the support. The hand nearest the toes will execute the twisting action. The two hands should be used as a unit, keeping all the fingers together and the two hands touching at all times. Keeping the support hand very steady, twist the working hand up and down. The support hand must remain completely stationary. Then move both hands forward slightly and repeat the twisting action.

Continue this movement (grip, twist, reposition, grip, twist, reposition) until you reach the neck reflex area at the base of the big toe. Do not twist both hands at the same time. Repeat this on both feet. If the person is tense it may be necessary to repeat a few times. This is a very effective technique for reducing tension.

WRINGING THE FOOT

This is similar to the spinal twist, except both hands move in the wringing motion. Grab the foot in both hands as you would a wet towel and wring gently,

LEFT WRINGING THE FOOT IS USED TO RELAX THE BODY FROM THE NECK TO THE BASE OF THE SPINE.

each hand twisting in opposite directions. Your elbows should fly up and move when you do this. Move the hands gradually up the foot to 'wring' the entire foot.

ROTATE ALL TOES

The principle here is the same as in the ankle rotation. It is a relaxation technique that not only increases flexibility of the toes, but releases tension and loosens muscles in the neck and shoulder line. The big toe is most important here. It represents half of the head area. The head joins the body as the toe joins the foot, so the area joining the toe to the foot corresponds to the neck. To execute this procedure begin with the big toe and work through all the toes of one foot before moving on to the

ABOVE ROTATING THE TOES MAKES THEM MORE FLEXIBLE.

107

other foot. Hold the foot with the support hand in the standard support grip. With the thumb and fingers of the support hand, firmly hold the base of the toe you are going to rotate. With the working hand, grasp the toe close to the base joint (metatarsal/phalange joint), with the thumb below, index and third finger on top. Now gently 'lift' the toe in its joint with a slight upward pull, and rotate in 360 degree circles, clockwise and anticlockwise, a few times. Movements must be gentle but firm, the support hand stabilizing each toe individually at the base as it is worked on.

SOLAR PLEXUS

The solar plexus is referred to as the 'nerve switchboard' of the body, as it is the main storage area for stress. Applying pressure to this reflex will always bring about a feeling of relaxation.

To locate the solar plexus reflex, grasp the top of the foot at the metatarsal area and squeeze gently. A depression will appear on the sole of the foot at the centre of the diaphragm line, which is at the centre of the base of the ball of the foot. This is the solar plexus reflex.

This technique is applied to both feet simultaneously. Pressure applied to this reflex is usually used as a relaxation technique to complete the treatment but can be used at any time during treatment if necessary.

ABOVE WORKING ON THE SOLAR PLEXUS IS AN IDEAL TECHNIQUE FOR INDIVIDUALS WHO SUFFER FROM STRESS-RELATED DISORDERS AS IT IS THE MAIN STORAGE POINT FOR STRESS.

Take the left foot in the right hand and the right foot in the left hand, fingers on top, thumbs below – from the outside of the foot. Place the tips of the thumbs on the solar plexus reflex. Ask your client to inhale slowly as you press in on this point and exhale as you release pressure. Make sure that you do not lose contact with the foot.

Repeat the solar plexus exercise a few times.

GRIPS

The following are descriptions of the specific or hand positions used in reflexology. They aid comfortable and effective execution of the thumb and finger pressure techniques.

GRIP A

Make a clenched fist with the working hand, keeping the thumb free. The fist of the working hand will provide additional support on the sole of the foot. The 'rotating

LEFT THIS GRIP IS USED TO WORK THE SINUS, CHRONIC EYE AND EAR, BRONCHIA, LUNG AND HEART REFLEXES.

thumb' technique is used to exert pressure on the reflex points. The support hand is in the standard support position, close to the working hand. With Grip A the left hand is usually the support hand and the right hand the worker.

REFLEXES WORKED WITH GRIP A

Sinuses
Chronic eyes and ears
Bronchia, lungs, heart

GRIP B

Here the support hand holds the foot in the standard support grip close to the toes. With the working hand, clasp the foot from above. Place the fingers on the top of the feet pointing towards the ankle. The thumb is then positioned to work under the toes.

REFLEXES WORKED WITH GRIP B

Pituitary gland
Brain matter
Eyes and ears

GRIP C

This is an alternative grip with which to locate and stimulate the pituitary gland if you have difficulty with Grip B. Bend the index finger at the second joint and use this as you would the thumb, find the reflex, press in, rotate

RIGHT THIS GRIP IS USED TO STIMULATE THE PITUITARY GLAND.

clockwise and anticlockwise a few times. Release pressure when you feel the reflex has been sufficiently stimulated.

REFLEXES WORKED WITH GRIP C

Pituitary Gland

GRIP D

Here, the left hand is the support hand and the right hand the working hand on both feet. 'Cup' the arch of the foot in the palm of the support hand. The thumb of the working hand provides extra support on the sole of the foot on the thoracic reflexes, and the index finger is responsible for the rotations on the top of the foot. Place the third finger on top of the index finger to enable you to exert greater pressure on the lymphatic reflexes. With the thumb on the sole and fingers on top, reach between the toes till the web between the thumb and index finger touches the web between the big and second toe. Reach as far down the top of the foot as possible with the fingers and, using the rotation movement as you would with the thumb, work point by point towards the webs. When you get to the webs, apply a

tight, pinching pressure on the webs as these are the most active lymphatic reflexes. Repeat this between each toe, using the grooves between the metatarsal bones as guidelines. Repeat this procedure on both feet.

LEFT THIS GRIP IS USED TO WORK THE UPPER LYMPHATIC REFLEXES.

REFLEXES WORKED WITH GRIP D

Upper lymphatics

GRIP E

In this grip the elbows move out and up into the air to facilitate the angle necessary to get right into the thyroid reflex. The thyroid reflex covers the entire area of the ball of the foot at the base of the big toe, but the most important part of this reflex is found in the half circle shape right at the base of the ball, almost 'under' the bone. To achieve sufficient stimulation, you must get right in to the bone at the base of the ball and press 'up and under'.

With the support hand, hold the foot in the standard support grip, which must be positioned close to the working hand. The fingers of the working hand grasp the foot from the inside of the instep, fingers on top of the foot from approximately half way down the big toe, and

the thumb poised to work the important half moon section of the thyroid reflex at the base of the ball. With the thumb, press in and up to get right to the bone and use the 'rotating thumb' technique to work round the half circle of the ball, up to the neck and then cover the section at the base of the big toe.

ABOVE THE THYROID, PARATHYROID
AND NECK REFLEXES ARE WORKED
WITH GRIP E.

REFLEXES WORKED WITH GRIP E

Thyroid
Parathyroid
Neck

GRIP F

To execute this grip effectively, the practitioner must be seated in such a way as to be able to swivel in his or her seat so as not to be working the foot 'straight on'. When using Grip F, always work the outside of the foot with the outer hand and support with the inner hand from the instep; and work the inner side of the foot with the inner hand from the instep and support with the outer hand. The pressure is, as usual, exerted with the 'rotating thumb'.

Imagine the foot divided in half vertically. The object is to work horizontally across both feet as if they are a single unit, using the imaginary vertical line as the point at which to swop working hands. This may sound slightly confusing at first, but it definitely aids a smooth and flowing technique for working the digestive area.

ABOVE GRIP F IS AN EXCELLENT TECHNIQUE FOR WORKING THE WHOLE DIGESTIVE AREA.

112

REFLEXES WORKED BY GRIP F

Liver/gall bladder

Stomach, pancreas, duodenum, spleen

Small intestine, ileo-caecal valve, appendix

Large intestine

Kidneys, adrenals, ureters

GRIP G

For this grip, the foot is cupped in the palm of the working hand, the sole of the foot resting in the palm, leaving the thumb free to execute the 'rotating thumb' technique. The support hand is in the standard support grip. This grip is used mainly for working on the sides of the feet – the spine and bladder on the inner foot and the knee, hip, elbow and shoulder on the outer foot.

RIGHT THIS GRIP IS USED TO WORK THE REFLEXES ON THE SIDES OF THE FEET.

REFLEXES WORKED BY GRIP G

Bladder

Uterus/prostate/ovaries/testes

Spine

Knee, hip, elbow, shoulder

113

EASY REFERENCE TREATMENT PROCEDURE

This step-by-step sequence describes the various techniques and grips in the specific order for a full reflexology treatment. This is the standard sequence I teach, and I have found it gives excellent results.

RELAXATION TECHNIQUES
Achilles Tendon Stretch
Ankle Rotation
Loosen Ankles
Side to Side
Wringing the Foot
Rotate all Toes

HEAD AND NECK AREA - THE TOES

Sinus from big toe to small toe – Grip A

Pituitary gland – Grip B or C

Brain matter – Grip B

Eyes and ears – Grip B

Sides and tops of toes – Finger Technique 2

Chronic eye and ear problems and eustachian tubes – Grip A

Upper lymphatics – Grip D

THORACIC AREA - THE BALL

Bronchia, lungs and heart – Grip A

Thyroid – Grip E moving to Grip A

Neck – Grip A

ABDOMINAL AREA - THE ARCH

Liver, gall bladder – Grip F

Stomach, pancreas, duodenum, spleen – Grip F

Small intestine, ileo-caecal valve, appendix – Grip F

Large intestine – Grip F

Kidney, ureter – Grip F

Bladder – Grip G

PELVIC AREA - THE HEEL

Pelvis and sciatica – Knead Technique

REPRODUCTIVE AREA - THE ANKLE

Prostate/uterus/ovaries/testes – Grip G

Fallopian tubes/vas deferens – Finger Technique 1

THE SPINE - THE INNER FOOT

Spinal Twist – Relaxation Technique

Spine from heel to toe – Grip G

OUTER BODY –
THE OUTER FOOT

Knee, hip, elbow, shoulder – Grip G

CIRCULATION/
LYMPHATICS –
THE TOP OF THE FOOT

Lymphatics, breast area, circulation –
Finger Technique 3

RELAXATION TECHNIQUES

Kidney and bladder meridians – Pinch Technique
Solar Plexus Deep Breathing – Relaxation Technique.

SELF-HELP AND FOOT CARE

CHAPTER SEVEN

TREATING YOURSELF

Self-treatment with reflexology can be awkward and arduous, but if you are willing to devote the time and energy, it is certainly worth the

effort. There are, however, disadvantages to self-treatment. First and foremost, the all important relaxation is impossible to achieve this way. Secondly, the vital energy exchange between subject and practitioner, which plays a major role in the success of treatment, is lacking, as you are both practitioner and patient. Self-treatment is, therefore, only useful as a means of preventative treatment, general health care and first aid treatment to achieve quick relief for a condition until you can arrange for professional treatment. It goes without saying that this form of treatment can never be as effective as the professional treatment you will receive from a trained reflexology practitioner.

However, for those who are willing and able to devote the time and energy to

LEFT SELF-TREATMENT REQUIRES DEXTERITY AND A WILLINGNESS TO DEVOTE TIME AND ENERGY TO YOURSELF, BUT IT CAN BE EXTREMELY REWARDING.

themselves, self-treatment can have many beneficial results. Self-treatment can be undertaken by anyone reasonably agile, who can comfortably sit cross-legged or raise a foot onto the opposite knee.

Comfortable seating is the first prerequisite. Sit on a chair, or cross-legged on the floor or bed with cushions behind your back. If you are aware which reflexes are out of balance, work specifically on those. If not, work calmly and gently through the whole treatment in accordance with the techniques and sequence described in chapter 6. You should be as relaxed as possible, with no tension in the legs. Remember it is difficult to assess your own reflexes accurately.

A full treatment will take approximately an hour, which may be a bit much for many to contemplate. However, treatment of appropriate reflex points can be used to relieve headaches, migraines, muscle aches and other temporary conditions. At the end of a treatment, always take the time to sit or lie back for approximately 15 minutes and relax with breathing techniques.

117

Foot Care Treatments and Products

CREAMS AND OILS
A therapist may apply herbal ointment or oil to stimulate circulation and relax the client at the end of a treatment. It is a good idea to pamper your feet in this way at regular intervals – either after a self-treatment or merely to relax and revitalize your feet. There are

LEFT IF APPLIED REGULARLY, NATURAL FOOT PRODUCTS WILL MAKE YOU FEEL PAMPERED AND KEEP YOUR FEET IN GOOD CONDITION.

numerous foot creams available on the market but it is best to use a natural herbal product, such as an aromatherapy oil or herbal cream, for their beneficial healing properties.

FOOT BATHS

Foot and hand baths can be prepared with dried herbs or aromatherapy oils infused in boiling water. Foot baths should be taken as hot as possible (but not boiling) first thing in the morning, on an empty stomach and they should not last for more than approximately eight minutes.

CHEMICAL FOOT SPRAYS

Chemical foot sprays should be avoided as they clog the pores and prevent the feet from being able to sweat properly. It is not a good idea to suppress the ability of the body to sweat through the feet since excessive sweating is an indication of imbalance and should not be ignored.

ABOVE A WARMING HERBAL FOOT BATH IS A RELAXING AND PLEASANT PART OF ANY FOOT CARE ROUTINE.

SHOES, SOCKS AND TIGHTS

Synthetic shoes, socks and tights should also be avoided as they increase the likelihood of sweating. Leather shoes will allow the feet to breathe unlike plastic and rubber shoes. Stick to cotton socks and tights for the same reason.

REFLEXOLOGY SHOES

These shoes have 'quills' that massage the feet and stimulate the reflexes while walking. Using these is not a replacement for reflexology, but is beneficial since they promote lymphatic drainage and circulation in the feet. These should only be used in moderation as exaggerated use can overstimulate reflexes and cause discomfort.

OTHER FOOT AIDS

There are numerous varieties of 'foot aids' available on the market today – reflexology mats similar to the shoes, wood or plastic rollers, brushes and electrically operated gadgets and all types of balls such as golf and tennis balls. As with the shoes, these aids help tone and relax the foot and increase lymphatic drainage and circulation but they should only be used in moderation to avoid overstimulation. However, these are only useful for maintaining good health, and are not effective in treating specific problems. None of these aids can be more effective than, or can replace, professional treatment.

When using any of the 'roller' type aids, roll them in a uniform way with an even, light pressure over the entire foot – the bottom and sides of the feet. No special emphasis need be placed on any particular reflexes. Apply this rolling therapy every day for approximately ten minutes per foot.

Many practitioners would advise you to steer clear of these aids on the grounds that no mechanical implement could replace the practised hand of a practitioner for sensitivity. It is important to remember that these aids give no clue to the differing state of tissue tone or allow for accurate reflex reading and reaction. They can, however, be useful as preventative and maintenance therapy.

ABOVE FOOT AIDS SUCH AS ROLLERS AND BALLS HELP TO TONE AND EXERCISE THE FEET. THEY ALSO INCREASE LYMPHATIC DRAINAGE.

A natural foot massage is probably more effective than any gadget. A walk barefoot on the beach or the grass brings the feet into contact with the earth and the energies that flow through it, and provides a revitalizing, energizing and natural massage.

VACUFLEX SYSTEM

Modern technology's contribution to reflexology is the VacuFlex System. The VacuFlex System is a vacuum system that is modernizing reflexology. By applying pressure to the whole foot at the same time, the VacuFlex 'boots' stimulate all reflex areas in just five minutes. After removing the boots, discoloration of the corresponding reflex areas remains for a few moments, providing an accurate visual diagnostic aid. People generally find the boots less painful than hand massage and children can be treated quickly and comfortably with this system. This system also includes the treatment of acupuncture meridians, stimulating them with suction cups. So it is a two-in-one idea, reflexology and acupuncture. The entire treatment will take about half an hour.

ABOVE VACUFLEX IS A QUICK ALTERNATIVE TO REFLEXOLOGY AS ALL THE REFLEXES CAN BE STIMULATED IN JUST FIVE MINUTES.

120

FOOT CARE

Having now seen that every part of the foot represents a part of the body, the importance of treating the feet with a great deal of care and kindness is obvious.

Regular washing and careful drying will prevent cracks developing. A pumice stone and creams help soften hardened areas. Problems such as corns, verrucas and athlete's foot should be dealt with and a chiropodist consulted for persistent problems.

Feet should be kept warm and comfortable at all times. There is a good reason for this. I am, at present, living in a warm, sub-tropical climate, and have numerous clients whose children suffer from runny noses,

ABOVE TO SOFTEN THE SKIN, USE A PUMICE STONE ON ANY HARD AREAS OF THE FEET.

sinus and chest problems and bladder weaknesses. In this climate the temperature is usually high outdoors, so air conditioners are commonplace. This results in constant movement between hot and cold conditions. Most children go barefoot, and a sudden drop in foot temperature affects the reflexes as well as the related organs.

REFLEXOLOGY AND OTHER THERAPIES

Reflexology is an extremely effective holistic therapy, the positive effects of which can only be further enhanced by any other holistic therapy, attitude and activity. Many different factors influence each individual and therefore his or her ability to assimilate and respond to the healing process. Some are in our control, some are beyond our control. In order to help offset the negative effects of conditions that we cannot control – such as the earth's gravity, the movement of the sun, moon and stars, global and social pressures, and climate – we should make more effort to alter those conditions that we can change. This may require some discipline and effort, but will be a great contribution to acquiring and maintaining perfect health.

121

Factors that we can change include diet, relaxation and exercise. Many conditions cannot be treated 100 per cent effectively unless modifications are made in diet. A good practitioner will usually enquire about diet and make some useful suggestions. Relaxation techniques will also

RIGHT REFLEXOLOGY CAN BE USED IN CONJUNCTION WITH RELAXATION TECHNIQUES, SUCH AS YOGA, TO PROMOTE A SENSE OF DEEP WELL-BEING.

be beneficial as an adjunct to reflexology treatment. These include Tai Ch'i, yoga, meditation, breathing and visualization techniques. Some form of more vigorous exercise such as aerobics, swimming, jogging and the like is also recommended.

As reflexology is a holistic therapy, it can be effectively and successfully combined with various other holistic/natural therapies. These include Bach Flower Remedies, herbal treatment, naturopathy, Ayurvedic medicine, homoeopathy, hydrotherapy, shiatsu or any other forms of massage, acupuncture and the Alexander technique. However, do not attempt to apply all the different methods together, as too much stimulation will have adverse effects.

CONCLUSION

Reflexology is expanding rapidly throughout the world. This is evidence enough of its efficacy and popularity. The main objective of reflexology is to help people attain and maintain a better state of health and well-being. It does not promise to be a magic cure-all for all people and all complaints. But there can be no question that reflexology has carved a respected niche in the realm of holistic healing techniques.

A human being is far more than the sum of his or her parts. Reflexology helps us to attune to our bodies and understand ourselves as part of a greater whole – to tune into the natural laws of the cosmos and work towards a more holistic approach to life, an approach that results in a balanced and fulfilled life.

Perfect health requires discipline and energy, but the effort pays good dividends. The choice is yours – a productive, peaceful and fulfilled existence, or a life riddled with pain, anger and disease. Remember the old yogi saying: 'Health is a responsibility.'

BIBLIOGRAPHY

Byers, Dwight C., *Better Health with Foot Reflexology*, lngham Publishing, 1983.

Connelly, Dianne M. PhD, M.Ac, *Traditional Acupuncture: The Law of the Five Elements*, 4th Edition, The Centre for Traditional Acupuncture Inc., Columbia, Maryland, 1989.

Gillanders, Ann, *Reflexology – The Ancient Answer to Modern Ailments* Gillanders, 1987.

Goosman-Legger, Astrid, *Zone Therapy Using Foot Massage*, C.W. Daniel Company Limited, 1983.

Gore, Anya, *Reflexology*, Optima, 1990.

Grinberg, Avi, *Holistic Reflexology*, Thorsons, 1989.

Hall, Nicola M., *Reflexology – A Patient's Guide*, Thorsons, 1986.

Reflexology – A Way To Better Health, Pan Books, 1988.

Ingham, Eunice D., *Stories the Feet Can Tell Thru Reflexology*, Ingham Publishing, 1938. *Stories the Feet Have Told Thru Reflexology*, Ingham Publishing, 1951.

Issel, Christine, *Reflexology: Art, Science and History*, New Frontier Publishing, 1990.

Kaptchuk, Ted J., *The Web that Has No Weaver*, Congdon & Weed, New York, 1983.

Kunz, Kevin and Barbara, *The Complete Guide to Foot Reflexology*, Thorsons, 1982.

MacDonald, Alexander, *Acupuncture – from Ancient Art to Modern Medicine*, Unwin, 1982.

Manaka, Yoshio M.D. and Urquhatt, Ian A. PhD., *A Layman's Guide to Acupuncture*, Weatherhill, 1972.

Mann, Felix Dr., *Acupuncture*, Pan Books, 1971.

Marquardt, Hanne, *Reflex Zone Therapy of the Feet*, Thorsons, 1983.

Marsaa-Teegurden, lona, *Handbook of Acupressure II*, Ginseng du Foundation, 1981.

Nightingale, Michael Dr., *Acupuncture*, Optima, 1987.

Norman, Laura, *Feet First*, Simon & Schuster Inc., 1988.

Russel, Lewis and Hardy, Bob, *Healthy Feet*, Optima, 1988.

Thie, John F., *Touch for Health*, T.H. Enterprises, 1973.

Wagner, Franz PhD., *Reflex Zone Massage*, Thorsons, 1987.

USEFUL ADDRESSES

AUSTRALIA
Heather Edwards
PO Box 766
Mount Gravatt
Queenland 4122
Tel/Fax:
617 380 779 34

BRAZIL
Ivete Maria Fagundes
Rua José
Emmendorfer 1674
89253000
Jaragua do Sul
SC Brazil
Tel/Fax: 47 372 1909

CANADA
Cecile Myslicki
70 Parkville Drive
Winnipeg
Manitoba R2M 2H5
Tel/Fax: 1 204 253
9735 375
Vacuflex only

Karen Nel
1951 Glenarie
Avenue
North Vancouver
V7P 1X9
Tel: 1 604 986 7121

GERMANY
Andrea Schippers
Domkeweg 23
37213 Witzenhausen
Tel: 49 5542 71463
(Vacuflex only)

GREECE
Sandra Barlavas
Kameikov 7
Rhodes 85100
Tel/Fax: 0241 73 015

ITALY
Alberto Carnevale-
Maffe
Via Procaccini 47
Milan
Tel/Fax: 39 2 311116

NETHERLANDS
Karine van Niekerk
Frankenstraat 31A
2582 SE Den Haag
Tel: 31 703 545 304
(Vacuflex only)

POLAND
Dariusz Ruder
UL. Pathowskiego 8/9
02/750 Warsaw
Tel: 48 22 642 6056

SOUTH AFRICA
Inge Dougans
PO Box 68283
Bryanston
Johannesburg 2021
Tel/Fax:
27 11706 4206

SWEDEN
Ann-Chatrine Jonsson
Varmlandsvagen 438
12348 Farsta
Tel/Fax:
46 8 942 485
(Vacuflex only)

UK
Valma Bradbury
44 Purfield Drive
Wargrave
Berkshire
RG10 8AR
Tel: 0118 940 2016

USA
Jill Tonkovich
2222 Kilkare Parkway
Pt Pleasant
New Jersey 08742
Tel: 1 732 892 7566

Index

127

DIPLOMA COURSES IN REFLEXOLOGY AND MERIDIAN THERAPY

INCLUDING

• THE STUDY AND APPLICATION OF REFLEXOLOGY •

• THE PRINCIPLES OF CHINESE MEDICINE •

• ANATOMY AND PHYSIOLOGY •

Courses are available at branches of the School throughout the world. Alternatively you can qualify through home study via one of the Distance Learning courses.

For a prospectus and further information on the Vacuflex Reflexology System contact:

The International School of Reflexology & Meridian Therapy

PO Box 68238
Bryanston
2021 Johannesberg
South Africa
Tel/Fax: 27 11 706 4206
email: vacuflex@iafrica.com
website: HTTP://www.vacuflex.com